MW00976621

Bridging the Gaps:

An African-American Guide
to Health and Self-Empowerment

Bridging the Gaps:

An African-American Guide to Health and Self-Empowerment

by
A. Maria Newsome, M. D.
Cleo Washington, J. D.
Lorenzo Hester, et. al.

Vincom Publishing Co.

Tulsa, Oklahoma

Unless otherwise indicated, all Scripture quotations are taken from the *King James Version* of the Bible.

Bridging the Gaps:
An African-American Guide
to Health and Self-Empowerment
ISBN 0-927936-92-5
Copyright © 1996 by
Dr. A. Maria Newsome
P. O. Box 753597
Memphis, TN 38175-3597

Published by Vincom Publishing Co.
P. O. Box 702160
Tulsa, OK 74170
(918) 254-1276

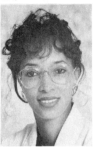

A. Maria Newsome, M.D.
Diplomate of American
Board of Internal Medicine

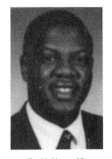

Cleo Washington, J.D.
Attorney at Law,
City Councilman

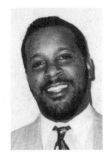

Lorenzo Hester
Businessman

Special thanks for the expertise of:

Rev. Celeste Williams
Associate Pastor/Adult Ministry
Mississippi Boulevard Christian Church, Memphis, TN

Howard Horn, M. D
L. W. Diggs Alumni Professor of Medicine/Cardiology
Univeristy of Tennessee, Memphis

Beverly Williams-Cleaves, M.D.
Associate Professor of Endocrinology
University of Tennessee, Memphis

Allen J. Hammond
Director of Student Financial Aid
University of Memphis, Memphis, TN

Cover Concept and Cover pages by **Peter Newsome.**
Artist and Advertiser

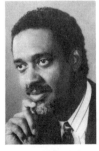

Melrose Blackett, M.D.
Fellow of the American College of
Obstetrics and Gynecology

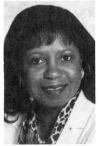

Loretta Bobo-Mosley, M.D.
Former Director Diggs-Kraus
Center for Sickle Cell Disease
Memphis, TN
Diplomate of American Board of
Internal Medicine

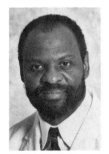

William Hurd, M.D.
Opthamologist

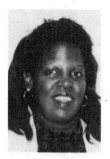

Robin Jones-Womeodu, M.D.
Assistant Professor of Medicine
University of Tennessee, Memphis
Diplomate of American Board of
Internal Medicine

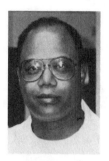

Kenneth Leeper, M.D.
Associate Professor of Medicine
Division of Pulmonary & Critical Care Medicine
University of Tennessee, Memphis
Medical Director of Pulmonary Medicine
and Respiratory Therapy
The Regional Medical Center, Memphis, TN

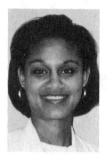

Yvette Randle, M.D.
Family Practice

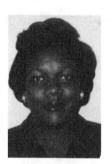

Delois Roberson, D.D.S.
Family Dentistry

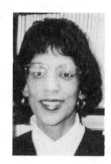

Yvonne Sims, M.D.
Fellow of The American College of Obstetrics
and Gynecology

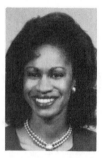

Rhonda Sullivan-Ford, M.D.
Obstetrics and Gynecology

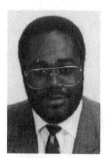

Ben Evans, M.D.
Internal Medicine

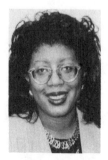

Carolyn Whitney, M.D., FAAP
Board Certified in Pediatric and
Adolescent Medicine

Dedication

Bridging the Gaps is dedicated to our Father God,
His Son Jesus Christ, and His Holy Spirit.

vii

Contents

Foreword

The African-American race has faced unthinkable hardships throughout centuries of racism and economic deprivation. Although many have prospered in spite of the obstacles, their numbers pale in comparison to the number of those barely making it, those "just getting by."

Masses of blacks still live in poverty, thus being unable to provide for themselves or their families in a comfortable, or even a safe, fashion. Many are unable to take adequate advantage of America's advanced health care system because they cannot afford regular doctor visits or prescription medicines, let alone health insurance. The suffering and death in the black community is disproportionate to the ratio of blacks in America. Countless numbers die each year due not only to inadequate health care, but also to a lack of understanding of their bodies and of the role each person must play in his own health and well-being.

Education is another crucial area of concern. A good education is more important than ever in a society where information is doubling in a matter of years. It is true that the black race has been ostracized and victimized many times over, but we must not allow the evil actions of others to define us.

We must be committed to educating ourselves and our children to be competitive in a capitalistic society. This means educational excellence, not mediocrity. It means "rolling up our sleeves" and joining wholeheartedly in the struggle to help other African-Americans realize their true potential, even if doing so will not directly benefit us personally.

During a Civil Rights banquet held in Memphis during September, 1995, author-playwright Eli Wiesel, a survivor of the Holocaust and a humanitarian, was very open about his refusal to hate his oppressors. He expressed a refusal to be bitter toward mankind because of atrocities committed during World War II.

He chose to love, forgive, and then work for the betterment of all men. His book, *Night*, which describes his ordeal during that period, leaves a reader amazed at his present gentleness and forbearance.

As a youth, he saw his mother and siblings separated from him — never to be seen again. He witnessed the cruel death of his father who had been dehumanized by starvation to skin and bones. Wiesel saw others of his race put into huge ovens to be burned to death, hearing their screams and smelling their flesh burning.

He witnessed many other demonic deeds perpetrated against multitudes of innocent people, yet he has refused to allow any outside events or forces to destroy his spirit, the inner man. He realizes that allowing those who hate you to dictate your behavior will ultimately destroy your mind and give your oppressor a double victory.

In some ways, this is what has happened with many African-Americans. By reacting to oppression and persecution with self-hatred, our communities now have self-destruction running rampant.

After consuming one's inner being, self-hatred spills over into acts of drug and alcohol addiction, violence against others, and socially deviant behavior. This is reflected in increasing crime rates and escalating high school drop-out rates.

As a race, if we refocused all of that negative energy into building one another up instead of projecting self-hatred onto other members of our communities, we would strengthen ourselves and our communities. We could break this apparent downhill spiral of self-destruction of African-Americans.

Instead of focusing on what other people have done and are doing to us, we need to focus on what we could be doing *for* ourselves — such as striving for academic excellence, supporting black businesses, and voting for those political candidates who best represent us.

Of course, centuries of racism will not be wiped out overnight; however, in the meantime, there are many things we should be doing for ourselves to lessen the impact of racism.

For example, if we had strong, black-owned businesses, hiring practices of racist companies would not have the potential to be so economically devastating. Unfortunately, blacks spend a very small percentage of their income at black-owned businesses.

It is easy to forget that the time was not that long ago when blacks were not welcome in many mainstream stores. Instead of appreciating the fact that we have achieved a certain amount of self-sufficiency and equality, we seem to have started to take it for granted. As a result of not being supported by their own communities, numerous black establishments are being forced to close.

This is not to say that blacks should not patronize stores owned by other races, simply that they should not neglect to support their own community stores as much as possible.

In the mid-nineties, as we see the political tide in America moving toward a more conservative stance, African-Americans need to be equipped to hurdle the obstacles that face us. To be empowered to weather the storms of life, we must believe in our own self-worth and in the self-worth of our race. We must be prepared to make strong, positive changes in our lives and in our communities.

This book is an attempt to provide some insight into

how we can become more self-reliant than we have been accustomed to being.

One factor that must be taken into consideration is the strong spiritual beliefs of our ancestors. Religion has played a very important part in the history of African-Americans and, unfortunately, in the rationale of prejudice against us as well.

Therefore, it is important to lay a foundation for self-help by pointing out the difference between biblical truths about blacks and the religious myths and traditions that have been used against us.

By dispelling these myths, we hope to establish the truth that the most important foundation of anyone's self-respect and self-esteem is *the eternal God*. Realizing that the Creator of all mankind (therefore of *all* races) loves all alike and is present with us always is imperative to understanding one's true potential.

The second thing this book attempts to do is explain, in lay terms, various medical conditions which affect blacks to a disproportionate extent. We give advice as to how each person can play a crucial role in his own health and life span, whether or not he presently has any medical condition.

The following chapters deal with self-empowerment through economics, politics, and education. Although there are many other gaps to bridge between the African-American and the other communities in our nation, we trust the material in this book will help the reader grow spiritually, physically, and economically.

The Authors

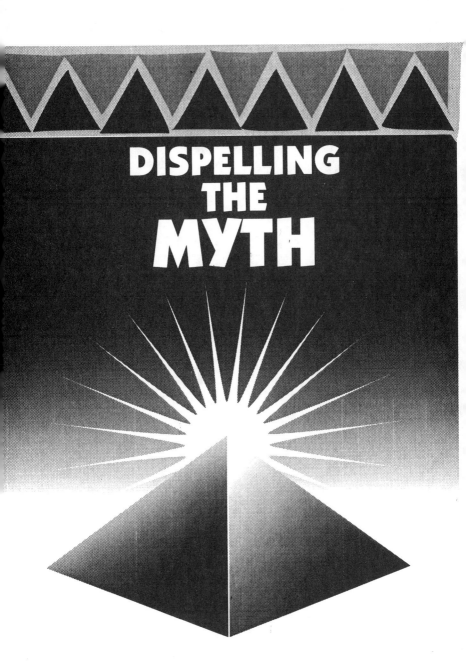

DISPELLING
THE
MYTH

The Myth of Ham

by A. Maria Newsome, M. D.:
Internal Medicine

Slavery, along with the unforgettable violence and cruelty that accompanied it, was sanctioned by the majority of Christians for years. In large part, this belief was based on an interpretation of the Bible that amounted to a biblical *untruth*: the myth of Ham's curse.

It was taught for centuries that God had cursed Noah's son, Ham, by turning him black and causing his descendants to be servants of the other races. Consequently, many felt it was the "God-given" right of Christians to enslave Africans.

The same "myth" caused Arabs, along with some other Islamic nations, to believe Allah sanctioned the enslavement of the black races. The Islamic nations were the first to target blacks for export as slaves on a massive scale.[1] Previously, empires such as Rome took slaves of conquered races, not just blacks.

Horrendous acts perpetrated against blacks after they were enslaved were justified as "putting down rebellion" or as "protecting one's property."

Unfortunately, too many Christians even today do not search the scriptures for themselves or read about the manners and customs of Bible days. Most simply accept what they are told by church leaders as "gospel" truth.

The fact is that we are obligated by God to check out what is told to us. (John 5:39; Acts 17:11; 1 John 4:1.) We are even to check what is told us by the five-fold offices Jesus set in the Church: apostle, prophet, evangelist, teacher, and pastor. (Ephesians 4:11.) We are not to judge those in the offices, but we are to measure what is taught or preached by the Word of God.

One good "rule of thumb" for judging is that if a purported Bible "truth" fuels pride, greed, or self-glorification, it probably is not a truth at all!

The majority of preachers are truly called, but it is up to them to renew their minds by the Word of God. (Romans 12:2.) Too many do not do this. Just as the people in the pews, they accept what they were taught and pass it on to others. No one is above error. Therefore, it is imperative for each Christian to read and study Scripture and develop a personal understanding of God's Word.

The scriptures that have been mythologized are to be found in Genesis 9, an account of what happened some time after the biblical flood. As only Noah's three sons and their wives are mentioned as being on the ark, this event had to be long enough after the flood subsided to grow and harvest a crop of grapes and for at least one grandson to have been born.

Ham is named in all of the early listings as the middle son: Shem, Ham, and Japheth. (Genesis 6:10, 9:19, 10:1.) In Genesis 9:24, he is called Noah's "younger" son but not Noah's "youngest" son.

Whether Ham was the middle or the youngest child, he is the only son mentioned as having a descendant of his own (Genesis 9:22) when the incident occurred that brought forth a curse from Noah. This is the curse that has been misinterpreted so badly.

The vineyard Noah planted after the flood had borne fruit, which had been made into wine. (Genesis 9:20.) Apparently Noah was not familiar with wine because, Bible scholars say, climatic conditions had changed so much after the flood. Before the calamity dropped so much water onto the earth, apparently fermentation did not take place.

At any rate, Noah became drunk and passed out in his tent. We are told that "Ham, *father of Canaan*," saw him and told his brothers, Shem and Japheth, who took a robe, walked backward into the tent, and covered up their father. (Genesis 9:21-23.)

That seems a small thing to bring forth a curse on anyone's descendants; therefore, there must have been more to this incident than is obvious. We can prove this by the original Hebrew words. The word for "nakedness" is the Hebrew *ervah*, the same word used in Leviticus 18 to refer to sex acts forbidden by God. It also means "shame or uncleanness."[2]

A different word, *aram*, is used in other places where the context is simply unclothed, as with Adam and Eve. (Genesis 3:7.)[3]

Three Lies Incorporated in the Myth of Ham

We have no way of knowing for certain exactly what was involved. However, in the context of slavery of blacks, there are three important things to see in the account of this incident. The myths are that:

1. *God turned Ham or Canaan black:* Nowhere in all the Bible does it say this curse involved changing the pigment of Ham's skin or of his descendants.

That "myth" is an assumption because those listed as Ham's children and grandchildren are also known in history as the progenitors of the brown and black races, such as Cush and Mizraim (Egypt).

2. *God cursed Ham and all his descendants:* Actually, only one son of Ham had a curse pronounced over his descendants, and the curse was from Noah, not God. However, most Bible scholars believe Noah was speaking prophetically from God.

3. *God cursed Ham's descendants with slavery:* The curse was on *one* son and his descendants only, and it was for Canaan's line to be servants, not slaves, in the tents of his brothers. (Genesis 10:24,25.)

To sum up: There was no curse to turn any of Noah's descendants black, nor was there a prophetic curse that *any* of them would be slaves.

The "bottom line" is that the Bible never puts down any race as inferior or superior to any other. The Israelites, later known as the Jews, were not chosen because of skin color or superiority, only because God made a blood covenant with Abraham, their ancestor and a Hebrew of Shem's line.

They were chosen for a purpose — to provide a spiritual line for Jesus and to make the truth of the one God known to the rest of the world. God Himself said they were not chosen because they were so great or so spiritual in themselves, but because He "loved their fathers." (Deuteronomy 4:37, 10:15.)

God chose Abraham because He knew this man would make sure the teachings about and worship of God would be passed faithfully down from generation to generation. (Genesis 18:19.)

When God calls, or "chooses" a man, group, or nation, it means they are chosen *to do something for Him*, not that they are picked as being special.

No Christian is chosen by God today under the New Covenant because of anything in ourselves, simply because we accepted Jesus. God loves us, just as He did Israel, because of our "forerunner" (Jesus) with whom He has cut a blood covenant. In fact, many are called but few are chosen, because those called will not always answer. (Matthew 22:14.)

Another real truth to be drawn from this story is that Adam and Eve are the parents of the entire human race.

Therefore, all earthly races had to be in and from Adam and none are more important than any other. Essentially, all mankind is related and are "brothers" in the natural sense.

Now that we have demythologized the color aspect, let us look at the actual curse of servanthood and see what that really meant.

Some think Canaan was Ham's oldest son, because he is the only one mentioned soon after the flood. (Genesis 9:25.) This would make sense in light of the customs of the Middle East in Bible times. The birthright went to the oldest son, as did the family blessing. (Genesis 25:31.) Likewise, any curse of family line fell on the oldest son and his generations.

The only possible reason for a younger son to be cursed would have been if he were involved in whatever went on, along with his father, Ham, which is possible. However, you would think that would have been made clear. On the other hand, because of the birthright/oldest son principle, Moses would have taken for granted that his readers would know why Canaan was cursed.

If Canaan was not a participant, Ham's oldest son would have been the one affected by any curse, just as Esau was when Jacob stole his birthright and blessing. Curses and blessings followed the lineage for generations. In Genesis 10, Canaan is listed last of Ham's sons, but that may not mean he was the youngest but that he had been "demoted" below his brothers.

Judah, Jacob's fourth son, was elevated to first ruling place after the oldest son, Reuben, also dishonored his father by sexual misconduct. (1 Chronicles 5:1,2.) The second son, Simeon, dishonored Jacob by his actions against Shechem, a Hivite, and his family (Genesis 34:24-30), and the third son, Levi, was chosen for the priesthood and priestly offices, taking him out of the birthright line.

John J. Davis, noted Bible scholar and professor of Old Testament history at Grace Theological Seminary, has written something typical of the view of most modern evangelical scholars:

> It must be emphasized that Noah cursed Canaan, not Ham. Popular (although totally misguided) exposition of the passage has applied the curse to the descendants of Ham and ultimately to black peoples, and concluded that the latter are inferior and doomed to servitude. This unsubstantiated interpretation, however, is utterly foreign to the text.[4]

Who *were* Canaan's descendants? Africans? Egyptians?

No, Canaan's descendants were the "ites" Israel found in the land when they took possession hundreds of years later. In fact, the land of Israel was first called the "Land of Canaan."

The "curse" was fulfilled during the one thousand years when Israel possessed the land. The Jebusites, Amorites, Girgashites, Hivites, Arkites, Sinites, Arvadites, Zemarites, and Hamathites who survived the conquest of Canaan became servants of the Israelites, "hewers of wood and drawers of water," so to speak.[5] (Joshua 9:21-27.)

Sidon, the only descendant of Canaan whose line survived as a separate nation, finally was mostly wiped out by Alexander the Great. Canaanite territory ran from Sidon to Gaza to Sodom. In fact, the residents of Sodom and Gomorrah were descendants of Ham through Canaan.

It is unfortunate that many people, even blacks, still believe this false information about Ham and the dark races so that a myth continues to have a great psychological impact on African-Americans and on how they are perceived and treated.

How can one truly have self-esteem and a sense of self-worth if he believes that God has cursed him through his race or color?

How can he find beauty in himself if he thinks God sees him ugly?

How can he respect himself when in his heart he believes he is not worthy of respect?

Proverbs 29:18 says, **Where there is no vision, the people perish.** African-Americans need a new vision to give vitality from within. The efforts of outside forces to keep blacks down are not nearly as devastating as the mentality of many blacks which keeps them from rising up.

Myths Believed Become Chains of Mental Slavery

The visible chains on wrists and ankles have been replaced by invisible chains on minds and emotions, which can be just as hampering. A person with invisible chains of any kind cannot live and work with self-confidence. A sense of powerlessness in being able to change his environment will cause him to give up before he even begins!

If these psychological chains of inferiority and inability stemming from the "Ham myth" are broken individually and as a group, there is no limit to how high the African-American community can rise. We cannot continue to allow the lies told by those seeking our destruction to alienate us from God.

God is not against us. He is for us. He means us good, not evil. (Matthew 7:11.)

Not only is the Bible overflowing with inspiring scriptures and stories of things God has done for earlier peoples, including positive stories concerning people of the Hamitic races. There were, and are, many descendants of Ham's line besides the Canaanites.

Moses married an Ethiopian woman — if not his first wife, then as his second. His brother and sister, Aaron and Miriam, were chastised by God for coming against Moses' authority because he had married this woman. (Numbers 12:1.)

Incidentally, the fact that Miriam was cursed with leprosy, becoming "white as snow," (Numbers 12:10) being interpreted that the white races are white as a curse, also is a myth, albeit not as widely known or believed as the Ham myth.

Other examples in the Bible concerning blacks from Ethiopia and other Hamitic nations show that these groups were not considered under a curse or inferior by Israel.

Also, remember that African-Americans are not descendants of Canaan. The majority of the Canaanites were either killed or merged through marriage with Israel or the nations which later took them captive — Babylon, Assyria, Egypt.

The closest descendants of Canaan today are the Palestinians, but they are the product of so much intermarriage with other races, particularly Arabs, that they are by no means "pure" descendants. They are the remnants of the Philistines and other coastal tribes who were not driven out of Canaan's territory after Israel conquered the land, and during ensuing centuries, remained there in towns and villages.

In Jeremiah's day, an official of Judah's royal court was Ebed-melech, an Ethiopian who saved Jeremiah's life. (Jeremiah 38:12,13.)

The first convert of Philip, mentioned as the first evangelist, was an Ethiopian official of the queen's court. (Acts 8:37,38.)

Rahab, the innkeeper who befriended two Israelite spies checking out Jericho for Joshua, is a Canaanite who achieved distinction in spite of Noah's curse on her forefather. She later married Salma or Salmon of the line of Judah, and their son was Boaz, the great-grandfather of David, from whose line Jesus came. (Joshua 2:1-22; Ruth 4:21,22; Matthew 1:5.)

Present-day Egyptians, descendants of Ham's son, Mizraim, have intermarried so much with Arabs that most people today have no idea of their original color or features.

Ishmael, Abraham's oldest son who was the father of the Arabs (from Arabia where they first roamed) had an Egyptian mother and took an Egyptian wife. (Genesis 16:1, 21:21.) Neither the Arabs nor the Egyptians, however, were of Canaan.

The concept that a race brilliant enough to revolutionize math and science with its mind-boggling pyramids was descended from the same founder as its cousins, the African races descended from Cush, is too drastic for many modern Americans to acknowledge. Many times ancient Egyptians are portrayed as white by the media, in spite of early drawings that clearly show the Hamitic connection.

God is the Creator of all nations and the Father of all peoples, nations, races, and classes. Any prejudice or hatred of one group of peoples for another, regardless of being based on religion, race, or social class, is not of God.

God Counts Only Two Races

In Jesus, all earthly races have become one heavenly race (Galatians 3:26-29), "descending" from the Seed of Abraham. All Christians are brothers and sisters in the Lord with a blood tie thicker than any earthly blood tie. Actually, God only sees two races: His family of children and all the others who make up Satan's followers.

In the New Testament, those two races were Israel (then known as Jews), the "people of God," and Gentiles, which meant "people without God." In other words, the two races always have been believers and non-believers.

There are only two heads of permanent, or eternal, races mentioned in the Bible: Adam and Jesus, the first man and the Second Man. (1 Corinthians 15:45-49.) Within each eternal race are represented all earthly peoples, nations, classes, genders, and races. (Revelation 5:9,10.)

Without a personal knowledge of Scripture, it is easy to be misled by those who are sincerely wrong as well as those who are knowingly wrong. It is tragic that, when Bible stories are told in America, somehow the implication is that all those heroes were white. Actually, whites are descendants of Noah's son, Japheth, not even of Shem.

The geographical boundaries seemingly settled by Noah's sons are: Ham, the African continent (which includes Egypt); Shem, the Mid-Eastern nations, not just Israel; and Japheth, Europe and, consequently, America.

The God of Abraham, Isaac, and Jacob also is the God of Asians, Africans, Europeans, Hispanics, and all other earthly races. All had the same Creator and the same original ancestor, Adam.

Racism based on supposed biblical principles is a lie, and the result of ignorance and prejudice, not Scripture. In fact, the Bible contradicts this kind of inequity. God's love is too magnificent for us to worry about trivialities of rank.

The African-American community of the United States badly needs healing today. The problems facing blacks are very complex and numerous, but they all have one thing in common: Not one of them is so deep, great, or powerful that it cannot be moved by Almighty God.

God can move obstacles as well as give us strength to endure them until they are moved. Whether it is a white man in a white hood burning crosses or a "brotherman" selling drugs "in the hood," God can fix the situation *if we pray and believe.*

Without prayer, John Wesley said, God will do nothing. The reason is because He designed His Kingdom to operate as a cooperative "family business" with Jesus as the "Head," and us as the Body. (Romans 12:4,5.)

God did not intend for the Body to run things by itself, nor did He intend for us to sit down and have to be dragged around by the Head, Jesus.

We pray according to His Word and His will, He tells us what to do, and we do it. Man was created to have authority over God's affairs on earth. (Genesis 1:28.) Adam gave up that authority to Satan, but it was restored to Jesus and delegated to His Body, the Church. (Matthew 28:18-20.)

Often, we do what we think is God's business without praying, and it fails. Or we do our business and ask God to bless it, and it fails. The right way is to make sure it is God's business, pray, and expect Him to bless His purpose and His will through us. God's "business" is for His children to prosper and be victorious over Satan, no matter what race, class, or gender they are of in earthly terms. (Luke 10:19.)

The tremendous psychological and economic impact centuries of racism have had on the black race can do one of two things:

1. Thrive so that the American portion of the African race is destroyed.

2. Be broken up bit by bit until no prejudice is left.

That choice is not up to politicians, groups, or organizations. That choice is up to God and to us.

God can restore the self-respect and self-love that is missing in so many African-Americans, if we pray and ask Him to fill us with His love. Only by giving God our whole hearts and then loving our neighbors as ourselves *with His love* can we eradicate prejudice and racism. (Matthew 22:37-39.)

He can warm the hearts of those who would hold us back.

He can give us favor with those who would oppress.

He can give us wisdom and knowledge, but most importantly, love. Love is the key that opens doors to happiness.

His love gives us joy and strength.

Our love for ourselves builds character, ambition, and determination.

Our love for our brothers of all races lifts up one another. When we become so busy building ourselves and each other up, we will not have time or desire to tear anyone else down anymore.

If enough African-Americans would commit to follow 2 Chronicles 7:14, we would see a revolution of love turn America around.

> **If I shut up heaven that there be no rain, or if I command the locusts to devour the land, or if I send pestilence among my people;**
>
> **If my people, which are called by my name, shall humble themselves, and pray, and seek my face, and turn from their wicked ways; then will I hear from heaven, and will forgive their sin, and will heal their land.**
>
> **2 Chronicles 7:13,1**

[1]Willis, John Ralph, Ed. *Slaves & Slavery in Muslim Africa*, Vol. One, (Totowa, NJ: Frank Cass and Company Limited, 1985), Preface, pp. vii-xi; (*The Times Atlas of World History* (London, England: Times Books Ltd., 1978,1982), "The Emergence of States in Africa, 900 to 1500," p. 136; Bohannan, Paul & Curtin, Philip. *Africa and Africans*, Rev. Ed. (Garden City: The Natural History Press, Doubleday & Co., Inc., 1964, 1971), pp. 261-277,287,288,295,296.

[2]Strong, James. *The New Strong's Exhaustive Concordance of the Bible*, (Nashville: Thomas Nelson Publishers, 1990), "Hebrew and Chaldee Dictionary," p. 91, #6172.

[3]*Strong's*, p. 91, #6174.

[4]Davis, John J. *Paradise to Prison: Studies in Genesis*, (Grand Rapids: Baker Book House, 1975, 1989), pp. 128,129.

[5]*Ibid*, p. 129.

PREVENTIVE MEDICINE

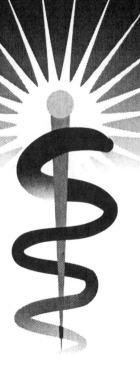

Health Care Introduction

by A. Maria Newsome, M.D.

The quality of health in the black community lags behind that in the white community for a number of reasons. Although financial constraints and access to care are important contributing issues, there are many ways in which the African-American community as a whole can actively participate in improving its own standard of health.

Learning about a variety of health issues can make a dramatic difference in a person's life by helping him to make informed decisions about his own life with a good understanding of the potential consequences.

Furthermore, utilizing preventive measures now can significantly increase not only the duration of life, but the quality of life. This further empowers a person to influence his own destiny.

The following sections were written by a variety of medical specialists in order to increase general awareness of common diseases that afflict African-Americans disproportionately. This knowledge is crucial to turning around the current health status of African-Americans.

Everyone should know as much as possible about any condition he or she may have. This involves asking questions of the doctor until a good understanding is reached. It is a good idea to write down (or have a doctor or nurse do so) the names of all diseases being treated, including those during a hospital stay, in order to have a *personal medical record* at home.

This may be a notebook with medical conditions, medications — what each is for, the dosage required, and how often to take it — results of important tests, advice given by the doctor, and the date and time of one's next appointment.

By keeping such a comprehensive personal medical record, a person can take an active role in managing his own illnesses. Also, he or she will be better able to communicate effectively with other health care professionals that may be seen later.

Also, it is helpful to keep a mini-list of these things in one's wallet or pocketbook, consisting of diagnoses and medications (with doses and frequency of administration). People often find themselves in emergency rooms or the office of a new doctor completely unable to explain their medical problems.

If a health care provider knows all of the illnesses a person has had, he can treat that person more effectively and efficiently. Of extreme importance is the fact that some medications interact with others in a potentially dangerous way. Still other medications may require gradual, not abrupt, withdrawal to prevent serious complications.

An issue not often dealt with among African-Americans is *organ donation*. Not enough blacks donate their organs. Tissue compatibility is very important in organ transplantation, and blacks are more likely to share similar genes with other blacks than with whites.

This means that, if there were a larger pool of organs from African-Americans, blacks needing transplants would have better chances of obtaining compatible organs and prolonging their lives. We need to seriously reconsider the rationale for refusing to let others live on through us once we pass from this earth.

The current state of health in the African-American community needs to be overhauled. In the midst of struggling for a better day for the race as a whole, we must not neglect those simple things that cost no money but can have a profound influence on our lives and the lives of our loved ones.

Our aim is not to make the reader a medical expert, but to give laymen basic understanding of common diseases and explain things that can be done to help prevent them from being as severe as they otherwise would be.

Hypertension

by A. Maria Newsome, M.D.

High blood pressure, also called hypertension, is a treatable, yet potentially deadly, disease. Each year it causes tremendous suffering and takes countless lives in America, and it affects blacks and whites disproportionately.

Not only is it more common among blacks, it is also more lethal. For example, for any given level of blood pressure elevation, African-Americans are more likely than whites to develop complications such as kidney failure.

Since the beginning of the National High Blood Pressure Education Program in 1972, great progress has been made in detecting and controlling hypertension. Along with an increased awareness and better treatment has come a substantial decrease in the number of deaths from heart attacks and strokes. Nevertheless, there is still a long way to go. Many people continue to suffer and die needlessly from this treatable condition.

One reason this disease is so deadly is that it often is "silent." Many people never know they have it until they find themselves in the hospital with one of its potentially life-threatening complications.

Still others are aware that their blood pressure has become elevated, but since they have no unpleasant symptoms, they do not want to spend hard-earned money on doctor's visits and prescriptions.

Ironically, the cost of controlling hypertension is negligible compared to the cost of treating its complications, which easily can climb into the thousands and even into the tens of thousands of dollars. More importantly, the needless physical suffering outweighs the financial hardships.

For example, when someone's kidneys fail, there are only two options left if he is to survive: a kidney transplant or life-long dialysis treatments.

If the person chooses a transplant, many issues must be considered. Furthermore, a compatible kidney may not even be available when he needs it. If one is available, are the finances available? The hospital bill for a kidney implantation may well be more than $50,000.

If a kidney is found and finances are available, this person must also consider the amount of time he or she is going to lose from work. Hospitalization might require several weeks, depending on potential complications. In addition, to prevent his body from rejecting this "foreign" kidney, the patient must take expensive medication to suppress his immune system the rest of his life.

In some respects, these "immune-system-suppressing-medications" place the transplantee in the same category as those with HIV infections, in that he will be at increased risk of developing a variety of potentially serious infections.

If the patient chooses dialysis treatments, he has three further options from which to choose:

1. Go to a center several times a week for a few hours.

2. Have home treatments that require self-motivation and a well-trained partner.

3. Have continuous dialysis by a cycle of infusing and draining dialysis fluid from his own abdominal cavity.

There are many potential complications related to end-stage kidney disease, including accelerated heart disease and hypertension, bone problems, infections and blood clots at the site of dialysis access, "dialysis dementia," itching, and poor nutrition.

Obviously, it would be better never to reach the point of kidney failure than to be forced to undergo treatment once it occurs.

Unfortunately, for reasons not clearly understood, black males tend to develop hypertensive kidney failure more often than others.

Hypertension Is a Major Cause of Strokes

Although kidney failure may cause a drastic change in a person's lifestyle, the most dreaded complication for most people is a massive stroke. This is one of the leading causes of death and disability in America, and uncontrolled hypertension is responsible for a large percentage of cases.

Although many people do recover partially, or even completely, a stroke has the potential to kill its victim instantly. Alternatively, it can render a person physically or mentally incapable of caring for himself.

Longevity is important, but most would agree that the quality of life is equally important. The abrupt change from being a productive, self-sufficient individual to being unable to work, walk, feed oneself, or possibly even talk, can cause emotional devastation as well as financial ruin.

Some people have multiple strokes involving several different areas of the brain which leave them paralyzed on both sides of the body, unable to control bodily functions, unable to think clearly, and unable to communicate. Yet, they are "alive."

There are two main ways hypertension contributes to strokes, known in the medical community as cerebrovascular accidents (CVAs):

1) The high pressure can cause a blood vessel to rupture, or 2) hypertension accelerates atherosclerosis, or "hardening of the arteries," which can (directly and indirectly) result in blockage.

In the first case, the stroke is a result of blood escaping its essential boundaries causing direct damage to brain tissue.

In the second case, a lack of adequate blood flow is the culprit.

Although they have different mechanisms and are treated differently, they have similar consequences. Fortunately, controlling high blood pressure substantially decreases a person's risk of having a stroke from either cause.

Blood vessels are similar to water hoses in that their walls actually have elastic properties and can expand to a certain degree. If a water hose carries water at a low pressure, it will last a long time. If water is forced through a hose full blast for a long period of time, the inside of the hose will wear down, predisposing it to develop leaks or even burst.

Similarly, when the pressure inside blood vessels stays high, wear and tear results, making their walls more likely to rupture. The small, delicate vessels of the brain are particularly vulnerable. When one of these vessels bursts, blood squirts out harming the sensitive tissues in the brain and causing a stroke.

On the other hand, a stroke caused by atherosclerosis is a result of the blood flow to the brain being blocked. Atherosclerosis plaques occasionally rupture and set up an ideal environment for a blood clot to form on top of them. If a blood clot forms on top of an already narrowed artery, it has the potential to completely cut off the blood supply, again resulting in a stroke.

If a blood clot causes the stroke, the patient is usually prescribed a blood thinner, such as a daily aspirin, when discharged from the hospital. Regular visits to a doctor following a stroke are very important.

Although kidney failure and strokes are responsible for much suffering and death, heart disease is still the number one killer in America, most of it due to the same complication of atherosclerosis (plague rupture and blood-clot formation).

The coronary arteries, which supply the heart, can be damaged just as the brain when the heart is deprived of blood flow.

Longstanding, uncontrolled hypertension frequently causes yet another heart condition called *congestive heart failure*. This simply means that tissues become *congested* with fluid when the *heart fails* to pump as strongly as it should.

This happens when hypertension causes the heart to get larger and larger. Because the heart is a muscle, it cannot contract very forcefully when it has been stretched too far, nor can it relax as well when the walls are too thick.

Symptoms of Congestive Heart Failure

A common symptom of congestive heart failure is a swelling of the ankles and legs due to blood vessels backing up "downstream" from a heart failing to pump "upstream" as it should. This is similar to a vehicle accident. Traffic behind the wreck becomes congested because it is not flowing swiftly. The blood cells themselves do not escape from the vessels, but fluid is pushed out under excessive pressure, accumulating in the tissues of the legs.

By the same token, another symptom of this condition is when progressively less physical exertion causes shortness of breath. When severe, the person may have difficulty breathing even when resting.

Furthermore, some people need to sleep on several pillows to prevent a smothering sensation felt when lying flat, because more fluid escapes blood vessels and moves into the lungs when a person lies down. Gravity layers out the excess fluid when one is lying flat. Consequently, fluid covers a greater surface of lung tissue. When this person returns to a seated position, this fluid falls to the bottom of the lungs and the person is able to breathe easier for a time.

However, there are other conditions that can cause the above symptoms. Therefore, no one should diagnose himself or herself as having congestive heart failure.

If you have any one of these symptoms, you should see a doctor for a thorough examination. Congestive heart failure is a treatable condition; however, it is potentially deadly.

As with all diseases and conditions, it is better to prevent it than to have to treat it!

Unfortunately, many people do not realize that uncontrolled high blood pressure can deduct many years from their lives. Death may be premature as in a massive stroke or a victim may suffer for years before slowly succumbing to congestive heart failure.

Other symptoms that may, or may not, signal the possibility of hypertension are:

1. Headaches in the back of the head, particularly in the morning

2. Lightheadedness

3. Dizziness

4. Heart racing

5. Chest pain

6. Nosebleeds

7. Ringing in the ears.

Medications and Side Effects

Any medication can have side effects.

If a particular medication does have an undesirable side effect, the patient may feel worse when he takes a dose than when he skips one.

Again, communication with one's doctor is essential because there is a very good chance of being switched to another medication that acts by a different mechanism. Unless there is a reason for taking a specific medication, a patient can often be switched to another drug.

However, it is possible there are situations in which it is simply not in the patient's best interest to switch medications. If side effects are minimal or likely to disappear over time, the physician may strongly urge the patient to continue using that medication.

For example, hypertensive patients who also have diabetes often are given a prescription from a class of drugs known as *ACE-inhibitors*. Certain Ace-inhibitors have a long-term beneficial effect on the kidneys of diabetics as well as controlling hypertension.

On the other hand, doctors often avoid a class of drugs called *beta-blockers* for hypertensive diabetics because they can mask the symptoms of low blood sugar, thus creating a potentially dangerous situation.

If side effects are intolerable or do not improve with time, the doctor certainly should be told. The doctor-patient relationship should be a partnership with mutual respect and understanding. A doctor should explain fully the pros and cons of any treatment so that the patient understands. After that, it is the patient who makes the final decision.

Although the initiating cause of high blood pressure is poorly understood, there are two major mechanisms that result in blood pressure elevation:

In one, the blood vessel walls constrict, increasing the pressure inside.

In the other, the amount of fluid inside the vessels increases with the same end result.

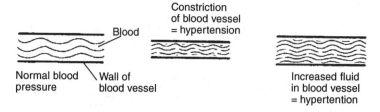

Complications of hypertension continue to wreak havoc, especially in the black community, mostly because of the widespread lack of knowledge about the importance of keeping one's blood pressure under control.

In some instances, instead of a lack of knowledge, problems result from a lack of good communication between a doctor and patient. Frequently, the patient feels too uncomfortable to tell the doctor that the prescribed medications are too expensive.

Fortunately, over the years, numerous medications with a variety of mechanisms have been placed on the market that are relatively inexpensive. Also, there are generic equivalents for many of the more expensive prescriptions that work very well for a fraction of the cost.

However, a doctor will not know to prescribe one of these if the patient is not honest about his or her economic situation.

The Effect of Salt on Blood Pressure

Most people have heard that excess salt in the diet can increase one's blood pressure. This is because the amount of water in the human body is directly related to the amount of sodium, or salt. The balance between the two is crucial. If one or the other is in excess, it can lead to serious consequences, even seizures and death.

Therefore, the body has receptors to gauge the relative

concentrations of salt and water and initiate mechanisms to maintain this balance. The kidneys are the final frontier for these changes. One of their functions is to alter the amount of salt and water being lost in the urine.

If water is the excess element, the urine will have more water than usual. However, if salt is in the excess, the kidneys will manufacture urine with more salt. By altering the urine composition, the kidneys are able to maintain the blood's composition in the normal range.

People differ in their sensitivity to salt. However, it has been documented that, as a whole, blacks are more sensitive to salt than whites. This means that, with a given amount of salt intake, blacks are more likely to retain water in the blood vessels, thus increasing the blood volume and, consequently, the blood pressure.

Many hypertensive patients take a "water pill" that makes them urinate more frequently, causing the body to lose more water through the kidneys. This decreases blood volume and, thus, blood pressure. The important thing to remember about these complicated mechanisms is that excessive salt worsens hypertension in many African-Americans.

Blood pressure is reported as two numbers: The *systolic* (sis-tol-lic) is the top number, and the diastolic (die-as-tol-lic) blood pressure is the bottom number.

When the heart is actively contracting and pumping blood into the blood vessels, it is said to be in *systole*. The blood pressure at that point is called "the systolic blood pressure."

Conversely, when the heart is relaxing and filling up again, it is in *diastole*, and the measurement is called "the diastolic blood pressure."

Normal blood pressure is considered to be approximately 120/80.

Borderline hypertension is 130-139/85-89.

Mild hypertension will measure 140-159/90-99.

Moderate hypertension runs from 160-179/100-109.

Severe hypertension is 180-209/110-119, and very severe is 210+/120+.

General Guidelines

Here are some general guidelines that are good for everyone to do, regardless of whether he or she already has been diagnosed with hypertension.

1. Have your blood pressure checked regularly, because hypertension often manifests itself as a person grows older.

2. If you smoke, quit! Cigarettes have a tremendous potential of worsening the outcome and shortening the life spans of those with hypertension.

3. Cut back on table salt (*sodium chloride*) and other forms of sodium in the diet. To do this, it is important to learn to read labels in the grocery stores.

Salt substitutes and various spices frequently can add as much flavor, if not more, to the food you eat. Although they often cost more than salt, the fact that using them may cut down tremendously on doctor visits, medications, and other medical costs makes them cheaper in the long run.

4. Purchase a book on nutrition, many of which contain charts or tables of the composition of a wide variety of common foods. Some even have the amounts of various ingredients that can be found in fast foods. Most people would be amazed at how much sodium they consume each day even if they never use table salt.

Gone are the days when we could just shop for taste and price. Content today is truly the most important issue.

5. As hypertension also speeds up the process of atherosclerosis (hardening of the arteries), it is especially

important for the hypertensive patient to keep his cholesterol level in the acceptable range. Reading labels and researching foods in nutrition books will help a person do this. We will discuss this in greater depth later.

6. Exercise regularly. Statistics show that, on the average, people who exercise regularly have a longer life expectancy than those who lead inactive lifestyles. Exercise helps lower blood pressure, reduce stress, and improves a person's cholesterol profile. Keep your weight down. If a person is overweight, losing those extra pounds may have a profound effect on the heart and blood pressure.

In summary, high blood pressure is controllable, although it is widespread and potentially devastating.

Considering the high prevalence of hypertension among African-Americans, all adults should have their blood pressure checked yearly *if* it has always been in the normal range. However, if a person already has shown some signs of hypertension, he should have his blood pressure monitored more often.

Take control of your blood pressure before it takes control of you.

Atherosclerosis/Coronary Artery Disease

by A. Maria Newsome, M.D.

Coronary artery disease is the leading cause of death in the United States as well as in most of the industrialized Western world. The coronary arteries are the blood vessels which supply the heart muscle with its required nutrients.

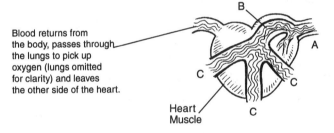

Blood returns from the body, passes through the lungs to pick up oxygen (lungs omitted for clarity) and leaves the other side of the heart.

Heart Muscle

The Heart and Its Arteries

Note that the large artery leaving the heart (A) gives off smaller arteries (B), which branch into additional arteries that supply the heart itself with blood (C). These last arteries are called "coronary arteries."

The main cause of coronary artery disease is atherosclerosis. Cholesterol, fat, and other materials combine to form hard, yellowish patches, called "plaques" or *atheromas*, which are laid down on the inner surface of arteries. With time, these plaques build up in layers, making the passageway through the arteries narrower so that less blood can flow through.

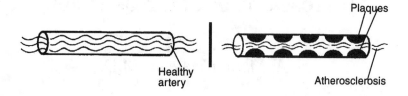

Healthy
artery

Plaques

Atherosclerosis

If this process is allowed to continue, the arteries supplying the heart can become so "stopped up" that very little blood is able to reach the cells of the heart. A drastic reduction in blood supply can lead to injury of areas of the heart muscle and even to death of that tissue.

Early in the course of this process, a person may have few, if any, problems. However, the more one exerts himself and the longer this condition continues to grow, the more likely a person is to know that something is wrong.

Exertion causes the heart to beat faster, and the more strenuous the exertion, the faster the heart will beat. When it beats faster, it requires more nourishment, just as a person becomes hungry and thirsty after a good workout.

If the blood supply to the heart is partially blocked, the heart will not receive all the nourishment it needs to function properly. As a result, heart muscle may be damaged. Reversible damage may manifest in the form of short-lived chest discomfort, called *angina*.

Early on, angina is often predictable because it may only occur with physical exertion. Less commonly, this condition may occur after a meal or a person's exposure to cold. Furthermore, angina can become so severe that it occurs even at rest.

Instead of severe pain, most people describe angina as a dull, squeezing or pressure-type of discomfort in their chests. Many have said it feels "like an elephant is sitting on my chest." This discomfort may radiate to the left shoulder or arm, neck, jaw, stomach, back, or even teeth.

There also may be accompanying shortness of breath, sweating, heart racing, nausea, or lightheadedness. Less commonly, a person may notice that when he exerts himself, he does not have any chest discomfort but does have one of the other symptoms.

As we will see in the next article, diabetics may not have any of these symptoms because of the nerve damage that is a complication of their disease. Furthermore, it is not impossible for people, especially diabetics, to have heart attacks due to blockage, but have few or no symptoms.

Other factors, in addition to diabetes, may increase the risk of heart attacks, such as hypertension, a *high* LDL cholesterol level, and cigarette smoking.

Consequences of Heart Attacks

As previously mentioned, the surfaces of the plaques may rupture and become rough, which increases the chance that a blood clot may form on top of them. This is where the "aspirin-a-day" prescription comes in. Aspirin is a "blood thinner," which decreases the odds of a clot forming.

When a clot does form, the already narrowed blood vessel can become completely blocked, causing a heart attack called a *myocardial* (or heart muscle) *infarction* (or death of tissue due to a deficiency of blood).

Complete blockage of coronary artery

Dead heart muscle due to a heart attack

More than a million heart attacks occur every year in this country. Of those, hundreds of thousands die before they ever get to the hospital. Of the survivors, tens of thousands still die within the first year.

Fortunately, the majority of heart-attack victims do survive past a year. However, many of these fortunate ones may continue to have problems long after the attack.

Unlike many tissues in the body, heart muscle does not have the ability to regenerate itself when it dies. After an attack, the dead area of the heart is nonfunctional and the heart loses some of its pumping strength. There are several possible complications of this situation.

A vicious cycle is set in motion because even less blood can get through the narrowed arteries when the pumping force of the heart has been compromised. This increases the possibility of later damage to living heart muscle and predisposes the heart to operate in abnormal rhythms, some of which can be life-threatening in themselves.

Congestive heart failure is another potential consequence of a weakened heart. Atherosclerosis of the coronary arteries causes the most deaths. However, hardening of the arteries in other parts of the body also can result in serious consequences, such as strokes, poor circulation in the legs and feet, which can cause severe pain or necessite amputation, or a form of kidney disease that can lead to hypertension.

Hardening of the arteries affects all parts of the body and can do great physical, as well as emotional, harm. Fortunately, there are some simple steps all of us may take to decrease our chances of developing these related conditions.

By understanding the major risk factors, we can make any needed modifications in our lifestyles to help us live longer, healthier lives. The major risk factors for coronary artery disease include:

1. Reaching ages of forty-five or older for men and fifty-five or older for women — early menopause lowers this age for women who do not take estrogen. (Estrogen is a female hormone that exerts a protective effect on the heart.)

2. Cigarette smoking.

3. Hypertension.

4. High LDL cholesterol or low HDL cholesterol.

5. Diabetes Mellitus.

6. Heart attacks or heart-related sudden deaths in fathers or brothers prior to age fifty-five or in a mother or sister prior to age sixty-five.

7. An inactive lifestyle and/or obesity are risk factors but not as significant as the first six.

Of course, age and sex are uncontrollable, but other risk factors can be controlled. These include giving up cigarettes, which dramatically increase the chances of having a heart attack; controlling one's blood pressure; getting regular exercise; making a serious effort to lose excess weight; and keeping one's cholesterol level in an acceptable range.

A Brief Overview of Cholesterol

One of the "building blocks" of atherosclerotic plaques is *cholesterol*. There are two main types: LDL (Low Density Lipoprotein) and HDL (High Density Lipoprotein).

LDL is the "bad" cholesterol. If it is elevated, a person has a higher risk of developing coronary artery disease than average. When HDL is high, there is a *lower* risk than average.

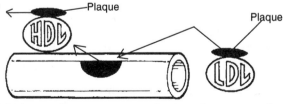

LDL brings plaques to arteries, and HDL carries plaques away from arteries.

According to the second report of the National Cholesterol Education Program, total serum cholesterol along with
HDL cholesterol should be measured in everyone twenty
years old and above at least once every five years. A patient
can have this done at a routine office visit, because this test
does not require any special preparation such as fasting.

For people without coronary artery disease, these
measurements apply:

Total Cholesterol	Class
Less than 200 mg/dl	Desirable Level
200-239 mg/dl	Borderline-High
240 mg/dl or higher	High cholesterol

HDL Cholesterol	Class
Less than 35 mg/dl	Undesirable: Associated with in-creased risk of heart attack
35 mg/dl or greater	Desirable

If a person has a desirable total cholesterol level, and
his HDL is more than 35 mg/dl, he simply needs to have his
levels checked at five-year intervals. This profile does not
increase one's risk for heart attacks. On the other hand, if
his HDL is less than 35 mg/dl, his risk for heart disease is
increased. This person should have additional bloodwork
done to break his cholesterol profile down further.

This is called a fasting lipid profile, done after no
food has been taken in for nine to twelve hours, generally
in the morning before breakfast. This profile gives the total
cholesterol, HDL level, LDL level, and triglyceride level.

(Triglycerides are another fatty substance that occurs
in the blood. Although they have less of an impact on heart

disease than the others, their level is needed to calculate the LDL cholesterol.)

Based on this profile, doctors tailor their recommendations to fit individual needs. Those recommendations range from simple lifestyle modification to daily medication.

Although the HDL level is a factor in determining overall risk, it is the LDL level that is the main culprit in heart attacks. Lowering a high LDL level has the strongest impact, although raising a low HDL does decrease the risk as well.

The desirable level of LDL is much lower for a person who already has coronary artery disease than for a person who does not. For someone with very few, if any, risk factors, the LDL goal is less than 160 mg/dl; however, if a person is known to have coronary disease, the goal LDL is less than 100 mg/dl.[1]

Quiz to test the reader's understanding:

Which of the following is the most desirable profile for a healthy individual without heart disease:

Total cholesterol	LDL cholesterol	HDL cholesterol
a. 295 mg/dl	220	70
b. 190 mg/dl	155	30
c. 198 mg/dl	138	55
d. 199 mg/dl	158	36

(Note: LDL and HDL do not equal total cholesterol as there is a small triglyceride factor that was omitted here for simplicity.)

Atherosclerosis is a long, ongoing process that begins in youth; therefore, a healthy diet is essential even in childhood. Furthermore, the eating patterns a person develops when he or she is young often carry over into adult life, at which point most of the hardening of the arteries occurs. (By the way, the correct answer to the Quiz is C.)

How To Lower Bad Cholesterol

By beginning screening as a young adult and making the necessary lifestyle changes, a person who otherwise would have been at high risk for having a heart attack as he grew older can be diverted into the low-risk category.

Even if someone has already had a heart attack, improving his cholesterol profile, if abnormal, can significantly increase his life expectancy. The first step in lowering bad cholesterol (LDL) is dietary modification. Important facts to keep in mind are these:

1. Cholesterol is only made by animals and humans. It is important for the production of hormones and other chemicals used by the body; however, the human liver makes enough to meet the body's needs. The liver manufactures cholesterol from saturated fat.

2. There are three major types of dietary fat: saturated, polyunsaturated, and monounsaturated.

3. The method of food preparation is very important.

4. Selection of meat used is crucial to diet modification.

5. Changing one's diet, exercising regularly, but continuing to smoke is undoing with one hand what you have done with the other. Smoking is the number-one *preventable* cause of premature deaths.

As only animals and humans have livers, cholesterol cannot be found in items that have no animal products. It is found in meat, dairy products, and other animal products.

It is *not* found in such things as vegetable oil, for example. Vegetables or grains or anything else outside the animal kingdom cannot make cholesterol.

Many advertisers take advantage of this little known fact by stamping "cholesterol free" on products that cannot possibly have cholesterol anyway. This leads the consumer to think cholesterol has been taken out as a service to the consumer and a good deed by the manufacturer. The label is true, but misleading.

Liver and egg yolks particularly are high in cholesterol. However, an occasional meal of liver will not do much harm, nor would scrambled eggs every now and then. As a better solution, some people make egg-white omelets and substitute two egg whites for each whole egg called for in a recipe. This will dramatically cut down on cholesterol.

The overall goal should be to have a good balanced diet, not necessarily to completely cut out high-fat foods. Therefore, when planning a meal, if one item is particularly high in fat, choose low-fat items to both prepare and accompany it.

For instance, when making a macaroni and cheese casserole, use skim milk instead of whole milk, egg whites instead of the whole egg, and low-fat margarine. That way, when cheddar cheese is piled on, the dish will still be much lower in fat and cholesterol than before. To lower the fat content even more, substitute low-fat cheese as well.

Since this dish would still be relatively high in fat, you might prepare lemon-baked fish or skinned barbecued chicken to go with it. Add a piece of wheat bread and green beans, and you have a delicious and nutritious meal. Even dessert can be low-fat or fat free, such as angel food cake, frozen yogurt, or fat-free ice cream.

Of the three types of fat, saturated is the worst by far, because the liver turns it into cholesterol. Monounsaturated and polyunsaturated fats are much less harmful. In fact, monounsaturated fat may significantly decrease LDL and total cholesterol. Good sources of this kind of fat are canola, olive, and peanut oils.[2]

The total daily intake of fat, however, should not exceed 30 *percent* of one's total caloric intake.

Recommended Breakdown of Daily Calories
Percent of Total Calories

Total Fat	Less than 30 %
Monounsaturated	10-15%
Polyunsaturated	Less than 10%
Saturated	Less than 10%
Protein	10-20%
Carbohydrate	50-60%
Cholesterol	Less than 300 mg a day

By getting in the habit of reading labels on food, a person can make a drastic improvement in his health. A product may boast of being cholesterol free but have a high content of saturated fat, for example. This product may do more to elevate the cholesterol level than a product high in cholesterol itself.

Learning To Read Labels Might Save Your Life

Many items say "reduced fat," but if their original product had a tremendous amount of fat and this product only has a great deal, again, the label is true but misleading. It will still likely have a negative effect on one's cholesterol level if consumed frequently enough and in sufficient quantities.

As heart attacks are the number-one cause of death in America, and the public now is aware of the health hazards of a high-fat diet, food companies have been forced to research and develop low-fat, or non-fat alternatives to traditionally high-fat foods. Some of these are very delicious and healthy, but truthfully, others leave something to be desired.

Pretty labels and fancy advertising do not make a product good for you. Look at how glamorous cigarette advertising has become. Regardless of all of the fancy packaging and enticing publicity, cigarettes are linked to hundreds of thousands of deaths each year.

Do not be seduced by the products of highly paid advertising agencies. They get paid to make their clients rich, not to help consumers live longer, healthier lives.

Learn to make your own well-informed decisions and do not be distracted by packaging or popular gimmicks. Most food items now *do* have a breakdown of the fat content.

All it takes to decrease the risk of dying from the number-one cause of death is a little bit of knowledge about processed and natural foods, determination to change one's diet, and creativity in planning menus and cooking meals.

Reading labels is more important even than comparing prices in order to save money. Is it not much more significant to compare labels in order to save lives, whether it is your own or those of loved ones?

Most labels list the total amount of fat along with the amount of saturated fat. Many also list the amount of either polyunsaturated fat or monounsaturated fat. Whichever is listed, if that amount is subtracted from the total, you have the percentage of the one not listed as well.

For example, if the total fat listed is 9 grams, and saturated fat makes up 4 grams while monounsaturated fat makes up 2 grams, then you know that the remaining 3 grams must be polyunsaturated fat.

Fat contains approximately 9 calories per gram.

Carbohydrates and proteins each contain close to 4 calories per gram.

All calories fall into one of these categories: Fat, carbohydrate, and protein. Obviously, gram for gram, fat is the most weight-producing food source. To give the reader some practice at reading labels, here is another hypothetical food label:

Calories	122
Protein	5 grams
Carbohydrate	21 grams
Fat	2 grams

Here is how to figure out the percentages, if they are not given:

Protein has 4 calories per gram, so 4 x 5 = 20 calories.

Carbohydrates have 4 calories per gram, so 4 x 21 = 84 calories.

Fat has 9 calories per gram, so 9 x 2 = 18 calories.

The total calories do add up to 122, but what is the *percentage* of calories from fat in this product?

To find out, the formula is calories from fat/total calories times 100 percent, or 18/122 x 100 = 14.8%. This product would be within the recommended guideline of keeping the fat percentage under 30 percent of total calories. The percentages of calories from proteins and carbohydrates can be found in the same way.

Keep in mind, this is only one item, and it is the *average* percent, not that of an individual item which is important.

A very common source of saturated fat in the diets of African-Americans comes from greens seasoned with chunks of animal fat such as pork "fat back." Although greens are very nutritious, they lose a lot of their overall health benefit when prepared with high-fat seasoning. Alternative seasonings, such as turkey slices or non-animal sources, would be more beneficial.

Other foods with a high content of saturated fat include dairy products and lard. However, most dairy products are now available in low-fat or fat-free varieties, allowing a tremendous reduction in fat but preserving the nutritional value. Instead of lard (from animal fat), vegetable shortening should be used.

Frying food adds a great deal of fat. Steaming, baking, broiling, and even barbecuing are better alternative methods of cooking, but beware of high salt barbecue sauces. Another hint about lowering fat intake is to trim excess fat from meat before it is cooked and drain off any fat left in the pan after it is cooked.

Low-fat or non-fat mayonnaise certainly ought to be substituted for regular mayonnaise, which is full of fat. Most Americans would benefit by cutting back on consumption of red meat and increasing the amount of poultry and fish in their diets. Fish, and skinless turkey and chicken are low in fat, but a hamburger is full of fat and sodium.

The Answer Is in Doing, Not Just Knowing

Now that we know how to reverse the trend of deaths from heart attacks, hypertension, and complications of atherosclerosis, it would be a tragedy if this does not happen. However, public awareness is crucial to any turn-around in these statistics.

Bookstores and libraries are full of material on how to lead longer, healthier lives. Radio, television, and magazines feature many segments and articles on fat-free living. Education and lifestyle modification will make a tremendous difference in stopping what amounts to an epidemic.

However, it does not matter how much information is available if people do not act on it as well as learn about it. If every reader put the suggestions in this article into practice, it would make a great difference in each life and in the African-American community as a whole.

Heart attacks do not have to remain the number-one cause that makes widows, widowers, and orphans! Do something about it in your own life and family!

[1]National Cholesterol Education Program Guidelines.

[2]Step 1 Diet recommended by the National Cholesterol Education Program for dietary modification.

Diabetes Mellitus

by A. Maria Newsome, M.D.

Diabetes Mellitus is another potentially serious disease affecting 2 to 4 percent of all Americans, yet it can be controlled. Contrary to popular opinion, diabetes begins more frequently in adulthood than childhood and is more common in blacks than in whites.

It is crucial for African-Americans to possess some basic knowledge about this disease in order to learn how to protect themselves from many of its potentially devastating effects.

The quality of life, as well as the longevity, of a diabetic can be improved substantially simply by learning a few basic facts. Furthermore, by recognizing the classic symptoms of this very common disease, an individual will be more likely to seek medical attention early.

Early treatment, which may only consist of certain modifications to one's lifestyle, is of a tremendous advantage in preventing several potentially serious complications. Countless people suffer from these complications which could have been prevented or at least delayed if they had only known more about this disease.

It would not hurt for everyone to learn the basics about diabetes mellitus in case it occurs later in life.

Another advantage of broadening America's understanding of diabetes is that more people will be able to help friends and family members who develop the classic symptoms. One who knows about this disease will be able to recognize it in others and counsel them to seek medical attention before their bodies are devastated.

Diabetes in its entirety is a very complicated disease process; however, the most important aspects can be explained in rather simple terms.

Our bodies turn much of the food we eat into a special type of sugar, called *glucose*, through a complex series of chemical reactions. This sugar then is transported into individual cells. Once inside the cells, glucose undergoes another set of chemical reactions that convert it into energy. This energy is used to carry out every bodily function from blinking the eyes to running a marathon.

However, many cells require a hormone called *insulin* to transport the sugar from the blood stream into the cells in order for the energy production process to begin. Insulin is manufactured by the *pancreas*, an organ that is located near the stomach.

When diabetes develops, it is because the pancreas is not making adequate insulin or because the cells are not responding properly to the insulin. In either case, the stimulus drawing sugar into the cells from the blood stream is diminished. Most of the sugar will remain in the blood stream depriving the cells of a vital nutrient.

In order to function properly, the human body must maintain a delicate balance of all the substances in the blood stream, as well as in the individual cells themselves. To ensure this balance, the body has very elaborate means of counteracting any abnormality.

For example, if the blood level of a particular substance is too high, the kidneys automatically filter relatively more of that substance into the urine in order for it to be removed from the body. This returns the composition of the blood back to normal.

In diabetes, the concentration of sugar is too high, and as most of the sugar cannot pass from the blood into the cells, it simply accumulates in the blood stream. Consequently, a lot of this excess glucose is filtered by the kidneys into the urine in an attempt to remove it and restore balance.

The problem is that, as the excess sugar particles are added to the urine, extra water is drawn in as well in a process similar to dissolving table sugar in tap water. Only so much sugar will dissolve in a given amount of water. Beyond that point, water must be added or the sugar will form a sludge. A similar process occurs in the kidneys.

In diabetics, the large amount of sugar in the blood stream is transferred to the kidneys, and as a result, excessive water is also lost in the urine. This is why diabetics have to urinate frequently. Their kidneys are working overtime making urine to get rid of the excess sugar.

At the same time, the body is losing so much water through urine that it must replace this water or dehydrate. The brain is aware of this need for water and responds by stimulating a sensation of thirst.

Finally, as sugar is being lost in the urine, weight loss can occur, as sugar is a primary source of calories. The brain telegraphs trouble in this case and sends out signals of increased hunger.

Because of this intricate process, classic symptoms of diabetes mellitus are:

1. Extreme thirst

2. Increased urination

3. Increased hunger

4. Weight loss

Other common symptoms include vomiting, nausea, blurred vision, tiredness, weakness, slow healing of cuts, numbness of hands or feet, frequent infections of gums, skin, or bladder, dry and itchy skin, stomach or leg cramps, a fruity odor to the breath, headache or dizziness, as well as frequent vaginal yeast infections in women.

See a doctor if you have any of these symptoms, although you may have another condition entirely.

Two Major Types of Diabetes Mellitus

There are two major types of diabetes, called Type I and Type II. All Type I diabetics require insulin, because with this condition, the pancreas makes little or no insulin. Type II is much more common, and insulin levels are decreased but not as severely as in Type I.

Type I is sometimes called "Juvenile Onset Diabetes Mellitus" or "Insulin Dependent Diabetes," because it usually begins in childhood. Although it can begin at any age, the typical age of onset is between eleven and thirteen years of age. Type I diabetics usually are thin.

More than ten million Americans are affected by Type II compared to about a million with Type I. The age of onset is usually after forty, and there is a stronger hereditary component than in Type I. These diabetics often do not require insulin shots, but the disease can be controlled with a combination of weight loss, dietary modifications, exercise, and sometimes, pills.

In some Type II cases, insulin levels may even be normal or somewhat increased. Unfortunately, this does not prevent the disease, because in these instances, the cells of the body that depend on insulin to transport glucose are not responding to the effects of insulin as they should.

Being overweight contributes to diabetes in most of the Type II cases. However, not all overweight adults develop diabetes. Obesity does render cells less sensitive to insulin. Therefore it is easy to see how being overweight could contribute to the onset of this disease.

In fact, Type II is so closely associated with obesity that many individuals do not become diabetic until they begin putting on extra weight. Fortunately for some, when they take off the excess poundage, their blood sugar levels return to normal.

Because of the relationship between obesity and diabetes, weight loss should be a top priority for those diagnosed with Type II and for those who want to decrease the risk of developing Type II diabetes mellitus in the future.

Even if a person still has diabetes after losing weight, the cells will not be quite as resistant to the effects of insulin, so this is a big step in the right direction. Although some medication still may be necessary, probably less will be required than before the weight loss.

In general, high fiber diets, low in fats and sweets, are recommended for a diabetic diet. Diet is of the utmost importance in managing diabetes. As a matter of fact, some people with adult-onset diabetes are treated solely with dietary modification and do not require pills or insulin shots.

However, even those who need medications also need to follow this diet with conviction. Therefore, it is critical for every diabetic to obtain a *Diabetes Exchange List* and learn how to use it. The following is a very short exchange list. Real exchange lists are *much* more extensive.

List 1	List 2	List 3
Starches/Breads	*Meat/Meat Substitutes*	*Vegetables*
Starchy vegetables		
Cooked cereal: 1/2 cup	Tuna in water: 1/4 cup	Greens: 1/2 cup
Cooked pasta: 1/2 cup	Egg: #1	Cabbage: 1/2 cup
Yams: 1/3 cup	Skinless turkey or chicken: 1 oz.	Vegetable juice: 1/2 cup

Plain popcorn: 3 cups   Lean beef: 1 oz.   Raw carrots: 1 cup

Potato chips: #10   Sausage: 1 oz.   Okra: 1/2 cup

Bread (white, wheat)
   1 oz. slice

Dinner roll: 1 small roll

List 4   ### List 5   ### List 6

Fruits   *Dairy Products*   *Fats*

Watermelon: 1 & 1/4 cup   Milk: 8 oz.   Mayonnaise: 1 tsp.

Medium banana: 1/2   Plain yogurt: 8 oz.   Butter: 1 tsp.

Raisins: 2 tbsp.   Hot cocoa from mix: Bacon: 1 slice
                             1 envelope dis-
                             solved in water

Raw apple: 1   Vegetable oil:
(Two inches across)   1 tsp.

Apple juice: 1/2 cup

List 7

Free Foods (Eat all you like of those with no designated serving size):

Celery, onions, green salad, salsa, hot sauce, radishes, coffee, tea, no-calorie soft drinks, lemons, mustard, water

Fast Foods

Wendy's Grilled Chicken Sandwich: 2 Starch/Bread, 3 Lean Meat

Taco Bell Regular Taco: 1 Starch/Bread, 2 Lean Meat

McDonald's McLean Deluxe: 2 Starch/Bread, 2 Lean Meat

[Note: The *serving size* is the number or quantity to the right in the lists above. For example, "1" serving of *fruit* may consist of 1 and 1/4 cups of watermelon, while "1" serving of *fat* may be a teaspoon of butter. When a meal calls for "3 meats" or "2 starches/breads," simply multiply this number by the serving size for "1" serving, and you will have the amount of a particular food that can be consumed at any given meal.]

For example, if you happen to be on a 1,500-calorie American Diabetes Association Diet, your schedule may look something like this:

Breakfast:

2 Starch/Bread (List 1)

1 Fruit (List 4)

1 Milk (List 5)

1 Fat (List 6)

Lunch:

2 Starch/Bread (List 1)

2 Meat (List 2)

0-1 Vegetable (List 3)

1 Fruit (List 4)

1 Fat (List 6)

Dinner:

2 Starch/Bread (List 1)

3 Meat (List 2)

1 Vegetable (List 3)

1 Fruit (List 4)

2 Fat (List 6)

Evening Snack:

1 Starch/Bread (List 1)

1 Milk (List 5)

Let's begin with a typical breakfast on this diet:

> 2 Starch/Bread (List 1)
>
> 1 Fruit (List 4)
>
> 1 Milk Product (List 5)
>
> 1 Fat (List 6)

Since you can have two choices from List 1, you might have 1/2 cup of cooked cereal and a 1-oz. piece of toast or a full cup of cooked cereal. You also can have one fruit item from List 4, according to our breakfast list. That might be 1/2 a medium banana, which you can eat by itself or add to your cereal. Then you can have one choice from Milk Products (List 5). You might choose an 8-oz. glass of milk or a cup of cocoa. Lastly, breakfast allows you one fat item (List 6), which could be a slice of bacon or a teaspoon of butter to go on your toast. (You may notice that some foods are listed under unexpected headings, such as "bacon" under Fat instead of Meat or Meat Substitutes.) Coffee comes under "Free Foods," so you can have all you want — without milk or sugar. Non-dairy creamer and a sugar substitute may be used.

Lunch and dinner may look something like this:

Lunch:	2 Starch/Breads (List 1)	McDonald's McLean Deluxe
	2 Meats (List 2)	(This would take care of both your first items.)
	0-1 Vegetable (List 3)	Green salad (which is free with a no-fat dressing)
	1 Fruit (List 4)	1 small raw apple
	1 Fat (List 6)	1 tsp. of mayonnaise on your sandwich
Dinner:	2 Starch/Breads (List 1)	2 small dinner rolls

3 Meats (List 2)	3-ozs. lean beef
1 Vegetable (List 3)	1/2 cup greens
1 Fruit (List 4)	1/2 cup apple juice
2 Fat (List 6)	1 tsp. of butter each for the rolls

These examples are only the beginning of potential meals. Each day, each meal may be different. Although remembering quantities and equivalents may seem difficult at first, over time these exchanges will become second nature. Dietary modification does not have to be boring or deprive you of your favorite foods. You simply need to know *how much of which foods* you can eat at any given time.

Ask your doctor to refer you to a dietician for additional counseling and obtain a more complete exchange list from either your doctor or dietitian, or contact the American Diabetes Association for additional information.

Every diabetic needs formal dietary counseling from a health care professional and should see a physician on a regular basis to monitor his condition. The patient may no longer require medication at some point in time if he loses enough weight, exercises regularly, and follows his diabetes diet.

Alternatively, the disease may grow worse and more drastic measures may be required. Even if the patient has been treated by lifestyle modification, diet changes, and weight loss, there may come a time when he needs medication as well.

Unfortunately, even when patients do see their doctors regularly, many times they will only take the prescribed medication when they are not "feeling well," especially if it is insulin in shots.

Exercise is almost as important as diet in controlling

diabetes. Not only does it help with weight loss, but it improves the ratio of body fat to muscle. Exercise can slow down the progression of the circulatory problems in the legs and feet that diabetics are naturally predisposed to developing.

Important tips for Type II diabetics include:

• Always follow the doctor's advice, even if you feel great. Do not "second-guess" his counsel.

If he wants you to keep a daily diary of sugar levels, do it!

If you smoke, stop it!

Limit alcohol consumption!

After all, it is *your* life the doctor is trying to prolong.

• Have your eyes checked at least once a year, because diabetics are more likely to lose their sight than non-diabetics, and there are treatments for diabetic eye disease.

• Have your blood pressure and cholesterol levels checked regularly, because diabetes increases the risk of having a heart attack. So make it a point to decrease any other risks over which you have control.

Exercise and Foot Care Are Important

Regular brisk walking is an excellent form of exercise for Type II diabetics. On the other hand, remember that diabetics are vulnerable to foot problems. They should wear "walking shoes" rather than ordinary tennis shoes. With any exercise, begin slowly *after* you have consulted a physician about your exercise program.

Foot care for the diabetic includes these important points:

1. *Never walk barefoot.*

Even stepping on a tiny pebble that has been brought

into the house might lead eventually to an overwhelming infection requiring amputation.

2. *Only wear well-fitting shoes.*

Shoes too big or too small cause irritations and subsequent skin breakages that could lead to infections.

3. *Examine shoes daily.*

Look over your shoes every day for any imperfections or loose debris that might cause irritations.

4. *Wash feet daily.*

Use gentle soap and warm water, then dry feet well. *Lightly* moisturize with lotion or oil, but rub it in well so the feet remain dry. Applying powder may help. Remember, bacteria love warm, moist environments!

5. *Keep feet warm.*

This will prevent drying and cracking of the skin. Avoid socks and shoes that cause feet to sweat excessively.

6. *Wear clean, soft socks that fit,* preferably cotton or wool. Your nails are softer after bathing, and this is the preferred time to clip them. Clip nails straight across and file the edges down with an emery board. Many diabetics have accidentally cut or scraped themselves while cutting toenails and have ended up requiring a foot amputation because an overwhelming infection would not heal.

If a toenail becomes ingrown, see a podiatrist (foot doctor). Also, do not perform even minor surgeries on your feet, such as scraping off corns or calluses or even bursting blisters.

8. *Examine your feet daily.*

Look for any signs of cuts or irritations no matter how small or insignificant they may seem. If you find anything, protect it at all costs until it heals.

For example, do not put your foot into a dirty shoe when you have a blister that could burst at any moment.

9. *Do not put on yesterday's socks or walk barefoot on your "clean floor" if you even have only a tiny cut on your little toe.*

If you do get a cut or a scratch, clean the affected area several times a day and completely cover it with a fresh bandage. Choose shoes and socks that will cause the least amount of pressure and stress to the area, and stay off your feet as much as possible.

10. *If any infection develops, seek medical attention.*

Indications of infection include any combination of localized warmth, redness, swelling, or drainage of pus (yellowish-white creamy material).

Go to a physician as soon as possible, and do not be embarrassed that you seemingly have such a "small" problem. If you wait until it becomes a "big" problem, it could cost you a foot.

Good foot care for a diabetic cannot be stressed enough.

Frequently, hardened blood vessels in the legs will keep enough blood getting to a foot to fight even tiny wounds. If an amputation did become necessary, poor blood supply might hinder the wound from healing well.

At this point, a patient could lose more of his leg to surgery in an attempt to reach a level where the blood flow is good enough to facilitate healing. Unfortunately, this is often somewhere in the thigh.

11. *Do not use heating pads, hot water bottles, or even hot water on your feet.*

Common Complications of Diabetes Mellitus

Twenty-five percent of all new cases of end-stage kidney failure are due to diabetes. This is the stage at which kidney function is not sufficient to sustain life. These people will require expensive, lifelong dialysis treatments or a kidney transplant, as we discussed in an earlier section.

Diabetes is the leading cause of blindness in the United States.

Atherosclerosis, or hardening of the arteries, can be another complication of diabetes. This can result in heart attacks or strokes, as well as diminished blood flow to the legs leading to extensive death of tissue. This is called *gangrene*. More than 50 percent of leg and foot amputations are the result of diabetes.

Damage to the nervous system is a complication not as familiar to most people as some of the other possible complications.

The danger is that when the nerves are not functioning properly, a person may not be aware that he or she has stepped on something sharp or clipped toenails too closely. Since the body's wound-healing capacity already is compromised due to diabetes, even these small injuries can lead eventually to amputations.

Alternatively, instead of being "deadened" or having their function lessened, nerve damage in a diabetic may manifest the opposite way. The sensitivity may be increased so that severe and chronic pain results, usually at night.

Another manifestation of nerve disease resulting from diabetes is paralysis of the nerves responsible for eye movements, swallowing, and the functioning of the digestive and intestinal systems. Also, numbness or tingling in the hands and feet (a "pins and needles" sensation) may be a result of nerves being affected.

In male diabetics, impotence (the inability to achieve or maintain an erection) is not at all uncommon.

There are other potential complications with diabetes as it can affect all parts of the body, but the ones discussed above are the most common.

If a doctor has prescribed insulin and not glucose-lowering pills, a person can take for granted that his baseline blood sugar levels are too high to be controlled with pills. Therefore, he ought to know that he will probably get into more trouble by skipping his shots than diabetics who skip a few pills — although no diabetic ought to take a chance by skipping any prescribed medications.

Another thing it is important to know is that stress increases the need for insulin. Even emotional stress sometimes creates a need for more insulin to control blood sugar. Diabetics should stay in close contact with their physicians, especially when ill.

A diabetic should never arbitrarily increase or decrease his own dose of insulin. This could throw him immediately into a life-threatening situation. Call the doctor if circumstances change in any way in your life.

The best way to "get a handle" on diabetes is to check blood sugar levels before meals and at bedtime. This check is much more accurate than urine glucose checks. Many people do not like pricking their fingers several times a day, but this is still the best means to keep diabetes under tight control. Once the diabetes is under good control, the frequency of these "finger sticks" usually decreases.

Structured sugar monitoring gives your doctor the best picture of where you are and facilitates the prescribing of medications and/or insulin more appropriately. The following examples illustrate this point.

Type	Onset of Action	Peak Effect	Duration of Action
Regular	15 to 30 minutes	1 to 3 hours	5 to 7 hours
NPH	2 to 4 hours	8 to 10 hours	18 to 24 hours

Many diabetics take a mixture of regular and NPH insulin in the morning and in the evening. We will assume this to be the case in the following examples.

Sample Table of Average Glucose Readings Over Time[1]

Time:		7 a.m.	11 a.m.	4 to 5 p.m.	9 p.m.
	a)	208	120	101	98
	b)	90	240	105	102
	c)	101	114	280	106
	d)	100	98	104	239

a) At 7 a.m., after "fasting" all night, the glucose is too high. This means the evening dose of NPH would need to be increased. Remember that the evening dose of regular insulin would have worn off by morning, but the evening dose of NPH would still be working, just not enough.

b) The glucose level before lunch is too high. In this case, the morning dose of regular insulin would need to be increased.

c) The glucose level before dinner is too high, so the morning dose of NPH needs to be increased.

d) The nighttime glucose level is too high, so the evening regular insulin would be increased.

Many physicians prescribe a combination of regular and NPH insulin to get more sustained control.

In addition, physicians sometimes give diabetics a *sliding scale* for insulin that tells them how much extra to give themselves if sugar readings do get too high. This allows the patient to take an active role in treating his own diabetes. However, this should be done *only* when the physician approves and oversees.

There are several types of insulin with different lengths of action. *Regular insulin* and *NPH insulin* are most commonly used. This combination is even available already mixed. It is called Insulin 70/30.

A few more points concerning diabetes ought to be mentioned:

• Diabetics are prime candidates for heart attacks that cause little or no pain because of the complications that affect the nerves and the arteries.

Even vague, mild chest pains or heaviness ought to be reported to a doctor. Any woman anticipating becoming pregnant should consult her doctor prior to conceiving. Proper medical advice and oversight will ensure the best possible outcome.

• Another common problem is when the blood sugar gets too low, because of poor timing of meals, too much insulin, or simply not eating enough.

Even non-diabetics can suffer from low blood sugar, such as when skipping a meal. In addition to hunger, common signs include sweating, shakiness, weakness, fast heart beats, feeling faint, headaches, confusion, and blurred vision. These symptoms are easy enough to correct — *eat something*, such as a piece of candy kept handy for such an occasion.

Every diabetic should be educated concerning his disease by a health care professional. Whenever possible, family members also should become informed enough to help out when needed and to spot any signs or symptoms signalling a potential disaster.

• Have a regular meal schedule.

In spite of all the potential complications, the disease is controllable. Nevertheless, millions of Americans have diabetes or will develop it during their lifetimes.

By possessing a little basic knowledge of the disease and exercising common sense, along with the advice of a physician, most diabetics can live normal, productive, and happy lives.

The best preventative remains watching your diet and your weight, but if you do develop diabetes, control it at all costs. By doing so, you may prevent blindness, kidney failure, or problems with your nervous system. These are well-established scientific facts!

[1]Greenspan, Francis S. and Baxter, John A. *Basic & Clinical Endocrinology,* 4th Ed., (New York: Appleton and Lange Publishers).

Preventing AIDS or Living Longer With It

by A. Maria Newsome, M.D.

Early in January, 1996, researchers from the Centers for Disease Control and Prevention announced that infectious diseases are now the third major cause of deaths in America, next to heart attacks and strokes.[1]

One significant reason for this rise is that certain strains of viruses and bacteria have evolved to resist most of the brave new drugs. However, researchers are working diligently to develop medicines to combat these organisms.

The death rate in the United States from infectious diseases rose 58 percent between 1980 and 1992.

Another factor involved in this drastic increase in deaths is felt to be climate change. Warmer winters, for example, have made places like Texas very attractive to the mosquito that carries dengue-fever, the cause of an epidemic in Latin America in 1995.

The main culprit, or the biggest cause of these deaths, of course, is the HIV/AIDS disease.

In 1981, the first cases of Acquired Immunodeficiency Syndrome (AIDS) were discovered, all of them among homosexual males. However, soon thereafter, cases began to appear in other groups, such as intravenous drug abusers, recipients of transfused blood products, and heterosexuals.

AIDS is caused by the Human Immunodeficiency Virus (HIV). The virus that causes AIDS is not genetically inherited, but is acquired by the mixing of blood or certain other body fluids.

It slowly destroys very important white blood cells that must be present to fight off harmful processes, such as infections and cancer, in the body. Once the virus particles invade the cells, they multiply over and over.

Eventually, the cells become overwhelmed by these particles and burst open. This releases these newly made viruses into the body at large, and they continue to infect and kill many more white blood cells as this vicious cycle continues.

Because the destruction of the body's protective cells is a gradual one, usually it takes years after being infected for a person to become seriously ill.

Once the virus has destroyed a sufficient number of the white blood cells, the person's immune system becomes deficient, thus the term *immunodeficiency*. As a result, the person becomes susceptible to unusual types of infections and cancers that normally do not make healthy people sick.

Many of these diseases are not normally strong enough to overpower a healthy body's natural defenses, so they are called "opportunistic diseases." They are like human opportunists who take advantage of the weakness of others for their own gain. However, if a person has a deficient immune system, these same otherwise harmless diseases can ravage his body.

The "S" in AIDS stands for *syndrome*, which simply means a set of symptoms that occur together. For example, the syndrome (or set of symptoms) made up of sneezing, runny nose, congestion, headache, and a general malaise (just feeling badly) occurs in the common cold.

The body of a person infected with HIV responds in the same way it would to any other infection, such as

HIV → ▼

The human immunodeficiency virus ▼ attaches to special receptors (Y) on the surface of special white blood cells called "CD_4 cells," or "helper cells" because they help coordinate the body's defense mechanisms

CD4 cell [or T_4 cell]
(a white blood cell)

The human immunodeficiency virus has invaded the CD_4 cell but initially remains dormant or inactive

Eventually, the virus becomes active (usually after a number of years). It multiplies over and over making many new virus particles

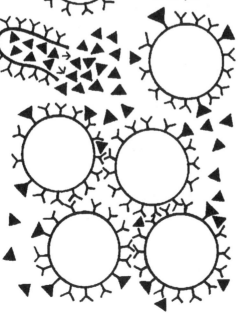

The viruses overpower the white blood cell and it dies releasing many virus particles which then infect new white blood cells, and the cycle perpetuates itself while it destroys more and more of these crucial CD_4 cells.

the common cold. The body produces proteins called *antibodies*. These proteins are the "warriors" of the body who fight against potentially harmful entities, such as bacteria and viruses that if not wiped out could cause disease.

Unfortunately, unlike many other harmful organisms that invade the human body from time to time, the antibodies are not strong enough to overpower HIV.

When a person is tested for HIV, he actually is being tested for the presence of these antibodies. If they are not present, the person is designated as HIV-negative. This means that probably he has never been exposed to this virus, or that his body has not had sufficient time to manufacture enough antibodies to show up in a test.

Most people with HIV within three months will have made enough antibodies to show a positive result on the HIV screening test, and by six months after exposure, the majority of infected patients will test positive. Therefore, someone who knows he has been potentially exposed but who has a negative test after six months can be pretty certain he does not have HIV.

On the other hand, if the time period since exposure has only been two months and the test is negative, it does not mean the person is "home free." His body may just not have had enough time to produce enough antibodies to produce a positive test.

Even before the test turns positive, a person with HIV can infect others!

The first test, called ELISA, is the initial screening test. If positive, the laboratory confirms the presence of HIV antibodies with a more sensitive test, the *Western blot*. Thus, before a person is told he is HIV-positive, his blood already has undergone two separate tests for the AIDS virus.

The Effect of HIV/AIDS on African-Americans

African-Americans again are disproportionately represented among those infected with this deadly virus, according to statistics of AIDS cases in America through December, 1994:[2]

Cases Among Black Adolescent & Adult Males		Cases Among Black Adolescent & Adult Females
Homosexual Males:	44,597	
Injecting drug use:	40,580	16,069
(Homosexual males who inject drugs — 8,479.)		
Heterosexual contact:	5,876	10,481
Hemophilia/coagulation disorder:	338	25
Recipient of blood or tissue components:	790	776
Risk not reported or identified:	10,298	4,470
Total:	**110,958**	**31,821**

These numbers only reflect those with AIDS, not those who were at that time simply HIV-positive. An additional 3,504 black children have been diagnosed with AIDS over the same period of time. This epidemic is devastating America, and the African-American community is being hit particularly hard.

When one considers the domino effect of transmission of HIV, it is easy to see how this disease has reached epidemic proportions in about fifteen years and how it will continue to spread *if attitudes and lifestyles do not change.*

Since it often takes years for a person to develop any

symptoms painful or annoying enough for him to seek medical attention, an HIV carrier can unknowingly infect many people through sex or sharing of drug needles.

In turn, all of those he or she infects can infect their subsequent sexual partners and/or contacts, ad infinitum.

It is easy to see how one individual could directly or indirectly infect many people over the course of several years. Obviously, the potential for transmission is mind-boggling.

Although there was once a time when heterosexuals in America were considered to be at low risk for contracting AIDS, this has changed dramatically. As a matter of fact, in sub-Saharan Africa, an area being hit extremely hard by this epidemic, heterosexual transmission is the major means of its spreading. However, as the statistics show, intravenous drug abuse is a more common source of AIDS transmission than heterosexual sex in the African-American community.

HIV/AIDS is a devastating dark cloud that is spreading its shadow across all racial, social, and economic lines. Before it is over, millions of Americans may die. It is crucial that each individual make intelligent, well-informed decisions in order to prevent contracting this virus.

Already, this epidemic has forced Americans to re-examine a variety of moral, personal, and religious issues. While those not infected need to understand this danger and make prevention a priority, we must not neglect or forget those already infected.

Ignorance breeds cruelty. Many AIDS victims today are ostracized even by their families out of fear and/or judgmentalism. Thus emotional and mental pain is added to the physical trauma through which they are going.

Everyone needs to know that not all body secretions have been reported to transmit the virus.

Urine, feces (bowel movements), saliva, nasal secretions, tears, perspiration, or vomitus are not considered means of transmission of HIV *unless* these secretions are contaminated with blood.

We do need to remember that it only takes one homosexual or heterosexual encounter, or one shared needle, to contract this virus. However, if every American who has engaged in one of those activities had contracted HIV, most of the country would be dead or dying!

AIDS patients do not need condemnation. If you have engaged in these activities and not become infected, then be very grateful and thankful. Do not let self-righteousness cover guilt and cause you to point the finger at those who have not been so fortunate.

Those suffering in this epidemic need love and support just as those with cancer or other fatal diseases. Over the next decade, numerous more men, women, and children will contract this deadly virus and each of them is someone's loved one.

Now is the time to purge the ignorance and try to bring emotional healing.

Now is the time to find out what to do to keep from contracting this virus.

At this point, there is no cure for AIDS. However, hopes are high that one day there will be a cure, and research is ongoing worldwide. In the meantime, everyone infected with HIV can take certain steps to improve the quality, and potentially the length, of his or her life.

AIDS Prevention

As the main methods of transmission are sex and drug use, obviously preventive measures must lie in those areas.

Sexual contact is the method through which most people acquire this disease. There are things everyone should do to protect himself.

First of all, abstinence until marriage and faithfulness in marriage are the best preventive measures. Unfortunately, in our society, comparatively few will do that.

Therefore, the next best suggestion is: *Never have unprotected sex.*

Having unprotected sex today is like playing Russian roulette or a game of chance where the odds are stacked against you.

Most people would not hesitate to turn down even a brand new Rolls Royce, if they were told the brakes could not be fixed and might fail anytime without warning. Every time two people agree to have unprotected sex due to inconvenience or potentially dulled sensations, they are playing a dangerous game of chance. Not just HIV, but unwanted pregnancies are a possibility.

Also, not all condoms are the same, so simply using any type of protection is not satisfactory. Latex condoms are preferable to natural skin condoms, which are more likely to leak the virus. Using a latex condom, along with HIV-inhibiting spermatocide nonoxynol-9 decrease the chances of contracting the AIDS virus even more.

Petroleum-based gels should never be used with condoms because they decrease their effectiveness against HIV. Also, even latex condoms may break or be used improperly. They are not even considered 100 percent effective in preventing pregnancy!

The only 100 percent deterrent in sexual matters is *abstinence.* The next best is a monogamous relationship in which both parties have tested negative for the virus after a six-month period of their last potential exposure, such as sex or a shared needle.

It is very unfortunate that many people go into denial when diagnosed with HIV. The impact is so traumatic that some people consciously or subconsciously refuse to accept it. Their denial of the situation is reflected in the refusal to alter their lifestyles. If they began to try to protect others, it would mean admitting that they have an incurable, fatal disease.

Some people consequently continue to infect others out of denial, or even out of anger and a desire for revenge. This is a childish, almost insane reaction. The people they will infect are not the ones responsible for the trouble in which they have found themselves. However, even with cancer and other potentially fatal diseases, human beings respond differently to the news of impending death.

Intravenous drug abuse is an even more common source of AIDS than heterosexual sex in the African-American community, despite the common belief that sex is the primary source. While the best option obviously is to stop using drugs altogether, many are so addicted that stopping seems impossible, short of entering a drug treatment program.

For those who are unwilling or unable to stop, the next best thing is always to use fresh needles and other "works" every time. And third best, for those unable to do even this, is to clean the needle or other paraphernalia after each use with household bleach and a thorough rinsing.

Blood product transfusion is now quite an unlikely source of contamination. The nation's blood supply is much safer now than in the past due to mandatory testing of all donors.

Individuals with HIV or AIDS ought to protect themselves and others who also have the virus fully as much as they need to protect those who do not have the virus. The reason is that different strains of the virus can be transmitted among those with HIV.

This transferring of strains could result in someone's contracting a strain resistant to certain medications that have been prolonging his life, thus accelerating one's decline.

Everyone not already infected should begin to take

preventive steps against becoming infected, and those already with the virus ought to be doing everything possible to improve the quality of life and to prolong life.

Nutrition may be one of the most important factors in this.

Malnutrition impairs the immune system and the ability to fight off infection in anyone, whether he has HIV or not. HIV-positive persons, in particular, should get established on a balanced nutritious diet. For some, vitamins or other supplements may be prescribed by their doctors to improve their nutrition.

A decreased appetite is common with AIDS, due to illness and medication side effects. If this is the case, eating smaller, more frequent meals often improves the nutritional status.

Chronic diarrhea is very common in AIDS, and this decreases the absorption of nutrients, making it imperative to get more nutrients into the body.

Regular medical checkups are crucial for HIV victims, even if they have not yet developed AIDS. There are certain stages at which different treatments should be instituted to improve or prolong life. Without consistent medical care, these stages cannot be recognized and treated.

For instance, HIV-positive persons who do get regular medical follow-ups may be started on AZT or other drugs that slow down the progression of the disease.

Checklist for Those With HIV Infection

• See your doctor regularly (at least every six months) so when your CD4 cell (T cell) count drops to various levels, you will be started on important drugs that have been proven to prolong your life. (A normal T cell count is 800 - 1,200.) Doctors often begin therapy with drugs directed at the HIV virus itself when the cell count falls to approximately 500.

NOTE: AZT is no longer the only drug that fights HIV. There are other newer, highly effective medications as well. *Do not miss the opportunity to get the best treatment possible. See your doctor regularly.*

• Have a tuberculosis skin test done as soon as possible after learning of your HIV status. You may need medication to try to prevent your developing active tuberculosis. Have this skin test repeated each year.

• Have a pneumococcal vaccine as soon as possible after being diagnosed with HIV. This vaccine may significantly decrease your chance of becoming extremely ill if you are exposed to the most common cause of pneumonia in the country.

• Have a blood test for antibodies to a microorganism called Toxoplasma when you are diagnosed with HIV. This helps to direct future prophylactic regimens.

• See your doctor regularly (at least every six months) so when your CD4 cell count drops to various levels, you will be started on important drugs that have been shown to prolong your life.

• Females should have two PAP smears in the first year after diagnosis with HIV, then once a year after that (cervical cancer is more common in those with HIV).

The following are common opportunistic diseases which occur during the course of AIDS in many individuals. By seeing a doctor regularly, important medication/preventive therapy, called prophylaxis, can be started at an optimal time which can significantly affect your life. Furthermore, your doctor may recommend a vaccine for Hepatitis B infection, or other interventions.

Opportunistic Infections and Prevention

In this section, I want to enumerate some of the more common opportunistic infections, some symptoms of these, and what prevention is known at this time.[3]

Pneumocystis carinii pneumonia, called PCP, is a very common opportunistic infection. As a matter of fact, most individuals with HIV will experience it at some point during their illness. Furthermore, it is responsible for a significant percentage of deaths in AIDS patients. Fortunately, there is effective treatment that will prevent, or at least retard, the development of this disease.

The common symptoms are fever, a dry cough or one which produces a slight amount of white sputum, pain in the middle of the chest (often sharp or burning) which often is worse when breathing in, shortness of breath on exertion such as walking, fatigue, and unexplained weight loss.

Adults and adolescents with HIV should receive pro-phylaxis against PCP in the following situations: 1) a CD4+ lymphocyte count of less than 200/microliter, 2) unexplained fever of over 100 F for at least two weeks, and/or 3) a history of oropharyngeal candidiasis, a fungal infection in the mouth that causes a white coating on the tongue, often called thrush. Note: Many *normal* babies also get thrush.

The best prophylaxis for PCP is *trimethoprim-sulfamethoxazole* (TMP-SMZ). For those who do not tolerate this sulfa drug, alternative drugs include *dapsone, dapsone plus pyrimethamine plus leucovorin, or aerosolized pentamidine* administered by the Respirgard II nebulizer.

Children born to HIV-infected mothers should receive TMP-SMZ beginning at four to six weeks of age. If the child is proven subsequently not to be infected with HIV, this medication can be stopped.

Toxoplasma gondii is an organism that commonly infects the central nervous system late in the course of an HIV infection. It usually is due to the reactivation of an in-fection that, until the immune system became severely compromised, had been contained by the body's natural host defense.

Many people are exposed to this organism early in life

and have no symptoms whatsoever due to this natural containment. However, the infection can become active later in life when the immune system loses its protective effect. Therefore, all patients who test positive for the HIV virus should have blood work done to look for the presence of antibodies to Toxoplasma, which would indicate prior exposure.

As stated previously, many people are exposed to this organism without their knowledge, and it is important to know if you have this organism in your body, even if it currently causes no symptoms.

Common symptoms include seizures due to brain masses, lethargy, dementia, coma, or weakness on one side of the body similar to a stroke.

To prevent exposure to Toxoplasma gondii:

• Do not eat raw or undercooked meat, especially pork, lamb, or venison. Cook meat until there is no pink inside.

• Wash hands after touching raw meat or soil.

• Wash fruits and vegetables well before eating them raw.

• If you own a cat, try to have a nonpregnant HIV-negative person change the litter box daily. If you are an HIV-positive or pregnant and must change it yourself, wash your hands thoroughly afterwards.

• Keep your cats inside, and do not play with stray cats.

• Feed your cat only dried commercial or canned food, or well-cooked table food. Use *no raw or undercooked* meat in its food. (You do not have to give your cat away.)

Indications that Toxoplasma prophylaxis is needed is a CD4 cell count of less than 100/microliter in those who have antibodies indicating previous exposure to this infection. Those who did not initially have antibodies to Toxoplasma should have this blood test repeated when their CD4 count falls below 100/microliter. If they have been exposed and thus developed these antibodies since their first blood test, they should receive prophylaxis.

Fortunately, all HIV-infected persons with this blood count should already have been started on PCP prophylaxis (when their cell count reached 200), and the doses of TMP-SMZ used are also effective for Toxoplasma prophylaxis. Therefore, no additional therapy is needed. For those who could not tolerate TMP-SMZ, the regimen of dapsone plus pyrimethamine plus leucovorin is effective. However, the other PCP regimens will *not* provide adequate coverage against Toxoplasma.

To prevent recurrences, those who have had a bout of Toxoplasma encephalitis (brain infection) need lifelong suppressive therapy to prevent a relapse. This therapy is usually pyrimethamine plus sulfadiazine plus leucovorin, or alternatively, pyrimethamine plus clindamycin.

There are no specific guidelines for children separate from those for adults. TMP-SMZ may be used during pregnancy.

Cryptosporidiosis is an opportunistic infection often contracted through animal or human feces, through pets or contaminated soil, or through swimming in contaminated water.

Possible modes of transmission include contact with infected adults or diaper-age children, infected animals, consuming contaminated drinking water, and through recreational activities in lakes, rivers, or public swimming pools.

To prevent contracting this, avoid contact with human or animal feces, wash hands thoroughly after any unavoidable contact such as changing a baby's diaper, wash hands after handling pets or contacting soil, avoid bringing an animal with diarrhea into your home, do not adopt stray pets, do not drink water directly from lakes or rivers, and avoid exposure to calves and lambs and soil from their farms.

Also, do not purchase a dog or cat less than six months old, or if you do, have a veterinarian examine the animal's stool for Cryptospiridium before having contact with it.

Be sure to boil water from your faucets at least one minute if there are outbreaks of cryptosporidiosis in your municipal water supply. No drugs have proven effective at this time at preventing this disease or its recurrence after an initial bout.

Tuberculosis cases have risen significantly since the outbreak of the AIDS epidemic, becoming widespread in America. Common symptoms include a chronic cough, unexplained weight loss, and drenching night sweats.

There are certain environments in which the incidence of TB is higher than others. These include homeless shelters, health care facilities, and correctional institutions, to name a few.

Persons infected with HIV should be aware of the increased potential for exposure if they live or work in any of these environments, or if they are in close contact with a roommate or friend who has active TB. However, they need not quit their jobs. They should consult their physicians to determine how great the risk is of contracting TB at their particular place of employment.

In fact, all persons with HIV should have a skin test for tuberculosis soon after they learn of their HIV status.

If this test is positive, and a clinical evaluation including a chest x-ray does *not* point to *active* TB — and if they never have been treated for or received prophylaxis for TB — they should receive a drug called *isoniazid (INH)* for twelve months. Pregnant women in this category should preferably receive TB prophylaxis after the first trimester. Usually, patients on INH also are given *pyridoxine,* a B vitamin, to decrease the chance of side effects on the nervous system.

Children of HIV-positive mothers should have a TB skin test at nine to twelve months of age, and those living in households with someone who has had a positive TB test should be evaluated. If children are exposed to someone with active TB, they should receive preventive therapy *if* active TB has been ruled out for them.

HIV-positive persons in close contact with anyone who does have active TB also should be on this preventive regimen. HIV-positive persons with a negative TB test should have the test repeated at least once a year. *Do not get a TB vaccine (BCG vaccine).*

After completing the treatment for TB, no chronic therapy is warranted.

Mycobacterium Avium Complex (MAC) is a bacterial infection caused by an organism which is ubiquitous in nature, and it can be found in soil, food, and water. Common symptoms include fever, night sweats, and weight loss. There are no guidelines at this time to prevent exposure to this bacteria.

A drug called *rifabutin* is initiated when the CDY cell count falls below 75/microliter. Patients who have had a bout of widespread MAC should receive lifelong therapy, usually with *clarithromycin* along with one of several other drugs. The same measures are appropriate for children as indicated for adolescents and adults.

Concerning pregnant women, there is inadequate data for a recommendation and the effects on the fetus of the drugs used in treating this are not yet known.

Bacterial Respiratory Infections include such infections as *streptococcal pneumoniae*, the most common form of pneumonia in America. In fact, these infections are so common, it is unrealistic to even consider preventing exposure to them. However, a single dose of pneumococcal vaccine should be given to all adults as soon as possible after documenting HIV-positivity.

Daily doses of TMP-SMZ, given for PCP prophylaxis, likely decrease the frequency of certain other infections. However, this drug is only effective against some of them. H. influenzae Type B vaccine is part of the routine immunization series for all children, not just those with HIV. The pneumococcal vaccine should be given to children over two years of age and to pregnant women.

Bacterial Intestinal Infections are more common in HIV infected individuals. Decreasing potential exposure is of the utmost importance, as prolonged or severe diarrhea has the potential to cause profound dehydration, wasting of the body, and even death.

The good news is that exposure to certain infections can be minimized by taking the following precautions:

• Do not eat raw or undercooked eggs or products that may contain them, such as certain preparations of salad dressings, mayonnaise, and hollandaise sauces.

• Do not eat raw or undercooked seafood, meat, or poultry. Be sure no pink remains in the middle after cooking.

• Do not eat unpasteurized dairy products.

• Wash produce carefully before eating it.

• Avoid cross-contamination of food, such as using the unwashed knife that has been used to cut raw meat to cut a piece of fruit. Wash any utensil used to beat raw eggs or cut or baste raw meat or poultry very thoroughly.

• Consider avoiding soft cheeses.

• If your pet has diarrhea, have the veterinarian check it for *cryptosporidium, salmonella, and campylobacter*.

• Wash hands thoroughly after handling pets.

• Avoid reptiles.

• Consult your doctor before traveling abroad, as the risk of diarrheal illnesses is increased in developing countries. Your doctor may want to give you antibiotics before you go.

• Persons who have had any of these infections and who live in a house or institution with HIV-positive adults, children, or pregnant women should be evaluated to prevent the perpetuation of recurrent infections.

Cryptococcal infection is another type of opportunistic infection that cannot be realistically prevented. Cryptococcal meningitis is the most common cause of meningitis (an infection of the lining of the brain and spinal cord) in persons with AIDS. It may also infect the lungs.

Common symptoms are fever, nausea and vomiting, headache, stiff neck, altered mentation (i.e., lethargy), cough, and shortness of breath.

One precaution that can be taken is to avoid pigeon droppings, which commonly carry this organism. To prevent recurrence of these infections, *fluconazole* is given as a lifelong treatment.

This therapy also is given occasionally to those with a CDY count of less than 50/microliter. Lifelong treatment to prevent recurrence in children is appropriate, but not mandated. Also, this drug should be used with caution for pregnant women because of its potential for harming the fetus.

Histoplasmosis is most common in people who live in, or have visited, the Mississippi or Ohio river valleys. Soil that contains droppings of birds or bats may contain many of these organisms. The infection may cause lung disease or may spread throughout the body.

Common symptoms include a fever of several weeks duration, weight loss, chronic coughing, and shortness of breath. As many of these opportunistic infections have similar symptoms, anyone experiencing them should see his physician.

There are no present recommendations for avoiding the disease. However, one can prevent exposure to these infections by avoiding activities that involve visiting chicken coops, caves where bats congregate, and other places where soil contaminants with bird droppings may be found.

Once you have had a bout of histoplasmosis, lifelong suppressive therapy with *itraconazote* is indicated to prevent a recurrence. The same is true for children who have been exposed to this infection.

Coccidiodomycosis is primarily a lung infection with most cases occurring in those living or visiting the southwestern United States. Again, common symptoms are fever, weight loss, and a cough.

To prevent exposure, avoid disturbed soil, such as on farms that are being tilled or in locations which have dust storms. There are no current recommendations for preventing the disease. However, there is therapy recommended to prevent a recurrence once someone has had a bout of this infection. That therapy is lifelong suppressive therapy, preferably with *fluconazole*.

Cytomegalovirus (CMV) is a viral infection common in patients with AIDS and can involve many parts of the body. Common symptoms include the painless loss of vision, "floaters" in the eyes, chest pain, pain upon swallowing, diarrhea, abdominal pain, weight loss, and a poor appetite.

There is currently no treatment recommended for preventing the disease. However, anyone experiencing "floaters" should see a doctor and should have regular eye exams called *funduscopic exams*. If you have had this, unfortunately, recurrences occur often, although chronic therapy with *ganayclovir* or *foscarnet* are of benefit.

The best prevention is to avoid exposure to this virus by:

• Using latex condoms, as CMV may be spread through semen or vaginal secretions. It may also be present in saliva and may be transmitted through blood transfusions, so only blood donors screened for this may be used.

• If working at a child care facility, good hygiene such as washing one's hands often, will decrease the risk of acquiring CMV.

Certain groups should have blood tests to determine whether there has been prior exposure to CMV.

Summary

AIDS is an acquired deficiency of the immune system, the end result of infection with the Human Immunodeficiency Virus, which produces a syndrome characterized by the presence of various opportunistic diseases.

It is primarily contracted by sexual contact, shared drug paraphernalia, or passed from mother to baby, usually during pregnancy. At this point, it is incurable, although intensive research is continuing all over the world in search of a possible cure or vaccine.

In the meantime, churches and community organizations need to "take off their blinders" and address this dilemma head-on before multitudes more become infected with this preventable disease. For instance, Mississippi Boulevard Christian Church in Memphis, Tennessee, has an AIDS ministry, the Healing Arms Program. It consists of an administrative/planning arm which plans fund-raising events, social activities, and a counseling arm for HIV-infected individuals who need these services.

In addition, several ministers in Memphis have formed an alliance, the African-American Leadership Consortium, which hosted the First Annual African-American Church HIV/AIDS Education and Leadership Conference in March of 1996.

Our communities need to be better informed about this epidemic, and the Church needs to take a leadership role in healing our land. Christ died for everyone, not just the "saints" who are "holy." After all, if human beings were capable of truly being "holy," Jesus would never have had to die in the first place.

[1]Centers for Disease Control (CDC), *HIV/AIDS Surveillance Report*, Vol. 6, No. 2, published in *Tulsa World*.

[2]*Ibid.*

[3]"USPHS/IDSA Guidelines for the Prevention of Opportunistic Infections in Persons Infected With Human Immunodeficiency Virus: a Summary," *Annals of Internal Medicine*, Vol. 124, February 1, 1996.

Respiratory Diseases in African-Americans

by Kenneth Leeper, M.D., FCCP:
Pulmonary and Critical Care Medicine

Deaths from respiratory diseases rose 20 percent between 1980 and 1992, according to the Centers for Disease Control and Prevention.

African-Americans make up 12 percent of the total population of the United States, and a significant number of them live in the central areas of our cities. This urban environment is responsible for the increased prevalence of several respiratory diseases in the black community, as well as in other minority group communities.

For example, black men make up a high proportion of the unskilled and blue collar work force, which means they are assigned to the "dirty" jobs involving exposure to dust and fumes that are risk factors in these diseases. Working in these jobs also brings a greater rate of decline in function of these men's lungs and a greater chance of lung cancer.

In addition to environmental factors, information is emerging from continuing research regarding genetic influences that may play a role in susceptibility of blacks to a variety of respiratory disorders. When the widespread use of cigarettes is factored in, we can see why these diseases affect more blacks in proportion to the population than whites.

Despite numerous studies documenting dramatic health risks for smokers, almost 50 million Americans continue to smoke — 28 percent of the male and 23 percent of the female population Smoking remains the leading cause of disease, disability, and premature death, killing more than 400,000 Americans annually.

Smoking is directly related to the development of chronic bronchitis and emphysema, two diseases that result in large numbers of diseases and deaths. Also, it has been known for fifty years that there is a connection between cigarette smoking and lung cancer.

According to a national survey involving large numbers over the past thirty years, it has been shown that African-Americans smoke more than whites, particularly males. Studies have shown that black smokers tend to use brands of cigarettes high in tar and mentholatum.

The danger of menthol cigarettes is that by providing a cooling sensation, they allow deeper inhalation. Consequently, more tobacco smoke is taken into the lungs.

Three common respiratory diseases are lung cancer, chronic obstructive lung diseases (emphysema and chronic bronchitis), and sarcoidosis.

Lung Cancer

Hardly anyone who reads or watches television does not know today that lung cancer is strongly related to cigarette smoking. Because of the high numbers of blacks who smoke, there is a higher incidence of death from this disease among African-Americans.

Of course, other factors, such as working in conditions that involve exposure to cancer-causing materials, add to the danger of smoking. A man with a smoking history who works in a plant where asbestos fibers are present is at a high risk for developing lung cancer and other cancers associated with asbestos exposure. Unfortunately, these cancers may not show up until twenty to thirty years after such exposure.

Nonsmokers exposed to asbestos have a five-times greater than normal chance of getting lung cancer, while smokers not exposed to asbestos have a ten-times greater risk. However, those who both smoke and are exposed to asbestos have a fifty-times greater risk.

Because the laborer positions in these unventilated factories (such as tire manufacturers) are filled predominately by black men, they make up a large portion of this high-risk group.

Chronic Obstructive Lung Disease

The frequency of emphysema and chronic bronchitis, however, is lower in blacks than whites. The reason for this is not yet known.

In *emphysema*, a majority of the air sacs in the lungs are permanently enlarged and their walls destroyed. Inhaled air is trapped in these sacs which press against the air passages causing obstructions. The primary symptom of this is severe shortness of breath, both at rest and upon exertion.

Chronic bronchitis is associated with an increased production of thick mucus that can block the air passages and be difficult to cough out.

Both of these diseases are progressive and cause severe respiratory decline and, eventually, death.

Sarcoidosis

This disease is not as well-known as lung cancer or other respiratory diseases, and it has the potential to affect nearly all the organs of the body, but quite frequently the lungs. It is a chronic disease of *unknown cause*, an inflammatory process which causes the lymph nodes, particularly those of the lungs, to enlarge.

It can affect the skin, eyes, and liver, but the most common symptoms are shortness of breath, coughing, and mild chest discomfort. While it occurs in all races and cultures, in the United States, sarcoidosis is ten to seventeen times more frequent in black Americans.

The disease usually occurs between the ages of twenty-five and forty and frequently is found in black women. In general, it is a rare cause of death. However, between the ages of fifteen and forty-four, the death rate among blacks is about twenty times that among whites. Also, black people are more likely to develop this disease in multiple organs than whites.

Patients with this disease must be evaluated frequently by physicians in order to monitor the course of the disease. The cornerstone of objective monitoring is lung-function testing which measures the degree of breathing function.

In about 70 percent of people who contract sarcoidosis, the disease does not progress and there is very little respiratory compromise. However, it can progress to severe lung disease.

If there is significant lung or other organ abnormalities, a physician usually will prescribe steroid therapy to slow or reverse the inflammatory process. Steroids have been found to be very effective against this disease, but they have their own side effects. Therefore, good communication between a patient and his physician is very important, in order that the effect of this medication may be continually monitored.

Asthma: Cause and Treatment

Nearly 14 million people in the United States are afflicted with asthma, and the numbers of those dying of this condition have dramatically increased over the past fifteen years.

The death rate from asthma has particularly increased in several large metropolitan areas, such as New York, Chicago, and Los Angeles. The annual cost for health care is estimated at $6 billion, with nearly half the costs going for emergency room and other unscheduled care.

Studies have shown that the urban environment appears to play a key role in the rising frequency of asthma. Various allergens, such as house dust mites, cockroaches, cat dander, environmental tobacco smoke, and industrial pollutants increase the frequency of this condition. These allergens often are responsible for the inflammation of the bronchial tubes that perpetuate the symptoms.

In all age groups, asthma generally occurs three times more often among blacks than among whites — especially in black children. Why is this so? Most experts say there are various socioeconomic factors that place black children at risk for this condition, according to several studies.

These factors include: premature birth, low birth weight, younger mothers, low family income which means living in large cities in inadequate housing conditions and asthma-causing environments, limited access to adequate health care, and underuse of anti-inflammatory drugs probably for economic reasons.

Black children also have a greater rate of hospitalization for asthma than white children. Asthmatic children of parents who smoke require more medication and have to make more frequent emergency room visits.

Medications that reduce inflammation in the lung's airways improve the long-term outcome of asthma. Specifically, *chronic use of steroid inhalers* has been found to be of benefit to most people with chronic asthma. However, it is important to know that these inhalers *do not improve symptoms during an attack.*

What steroid inhalers do is to decrease the frequency and severity of attacks and help preserve lung function. They should be used daily with the exact frequency depending on the specific medication. They should be taken whether or not a person shows symptoms of an attack, as they are preventives more than cures.

As the steroid is being applied directly to only one part of the body — the lungs — there is not going to be a significant effect on the rest of the body, unlike the situation where someone takes steroid pills on a regular basis.

However, in some cases of very severe asthma, a doctor may prescribe long-term steroid pills because of their increased potency. Each patient should discuss the use of these inhalers with a physician.

All asthmatics should obtain a *peak flow meter* from a pharmacy and learn how to use it. By blowing into these meters, a person can get an idea of how bad an attack is and phone his physician early on for treatment rather than ending up in the emergency room.

A physician may phone a prescription to the patient's pharmacy for oral steroids to be taken a limited number of days in such attacks. By so doing, potentially severe attacks can be stopped before they lead to disaster.

The patient then can visit the doctor as soon as possible to be checked out, eliminating the need for a fast emergency room trip. Of course, the doctor may give a patient a prescription for these pills to keep at home in case they are needed, in which case, he will want to be called before the patient starts on the pills to be kept abreast of the patient's condition.

Another important thing to know about steroid inhalers is how to use them. The technique for their use is crucial. Many people do not use the inhalers properly, so an appropriate amount of medication is not delivered to their lungs.

Two recommended techniques are as follows:

1. Put the inhaler between your closed lips, then activate it by pushing down on the canister. Breathe in and hold for ten seconds; exhale.

2. Open your mouth, but place the mouthpiece about one and a half inches in front of your lips, not in your mouth. Pump the inhaler at the beginning of a five-second inspiration (breathing in). Then hold your breath for an additional ten seconds before exhaling.

The second method is preferred over the first because it usually delivers more medicine to the lungs. However, some people have difficulty mastering either technique.

If so, they may purchase a device called a *spacer* from a pharmacy. Spacers can be invaluable aids in the treatment of asthma by making it easier to deliver the medication to the right place and in a sufficient amount.

Even with the use of a spacer, an asthmatic should take his inhaler to his doctor's office on a periodic basis to demonstrate how he or she uses it. If the technique is inadequate, the doctor can correct it.

As important as proper treatment of asthma is the prevention of attacks. In some cases, modifications around the home can sometimes make a significant difference. Carpeting traps a lot of allergens, so hard floors kept very clean probably are better for asthmatics than carpeted floors.

The right kind of mattresses and pillows, as well as sheets and pillowcases, also can help prevent attacks. Eliminate feather pillows, old pillows and mattresses, and items made of cotton and any other allergy-known materials. Air filters that remove dust and pollutants also can help.

It goes without saying that asthmatics should probably stay away from animals they know seem to cause flare-ups. Asthma does not need to claim as many lives as it does.

Regular visits to a physician and educating oneself about general maintenance, treatment, and warning signs of an attack can alleviate much of the discomfort and trauma of this disease.

In conclusion, black Americans are at greater risk of suffering and death from respiratory diseases, such as lung cancer, compared to whites. This apparently is because of the high prevalence of smoking habits in the African-American population, combined with factors such as poverty, environmental exposure to conditions that cause respiratory diseases, and low access to health care.

References

1. Coutlas, D. B., Gong H. Jr., Grad R, "Respiratory Disease in Minorities of the United States," *American Journal of Respiratory Critical Care Medicine*, 1994; 149: S93-S131.

2. Byrd W., Clayton L. "An American Health Dilemma: A History of Blacks in the Health System," *Journal of the National Medical Association*, 1992; 84: pp. 717-725.

3. "Black-White Disparities in Health Care," Council on Ethical and Judicial Affairs, *Journal of the American Medical Association*, 1990; 263: pp. 2344-2346.

Drugs, Alcohol, and Nicotine:
The Effects of Illicit Drug Use
Alcohol Abuse
Cigarette Smoking

The Effects of Illicit Drug Use

by Robin J. Womeodu, M.D.:
Internal Medicine

Introduction

Illicit drug use is a major societal concern that destroys the lives of individuals and initiates a cascade of problems for families, neighborhoods, and the community at large. Surveys have found that 21 million Americans have used cocaine at least once, and 21 million also reported using marijuana in the past year.

Among high school seniors, almost 44 percent report having tried marijuana and 10 percent report having used cocaine. Some people feel these data may greatly underestimate the problem because high risk youth who have dropped out of school are not included.

Using available data, it has been estimated that one in four American adolescents is at a very high risk of alcohol and other drug problems and their consequences. Drug use has been linked to high rates of violent crime, to transmission of HIV, to traumatic injuries from traffic accidents and falls, to serious medical conditions such as heart attacks and strokes, and to developmental problems in infants.

Cocaine: This drug is only one of many illicit substances; yet, in the last decade, its use has increased dramatically. The first mentioned use of cocaine dates back to 3000 B.C., but in the 1980s, the development of "crack cocaine" introduced a highly addictive, relatively inexpensive form of the drug that can be smoked. Smoking results in very high peak concentrations of the drug absorbed through numerous blood vessels in the lungs.

This form of the drug has resulted in a marked increase in medical, economic, and social complications. Cocaine use has been associated with many serious medical complications, including sudden death. The dosage that turns out to be lethal varies widely from person to person. Sudden death from cocaine is thought to be related to heart problems, seizures, respiratory arrest (the lungs fail), or strokes.

Cocaine use also has been associated with psychiatric complications such as psychosis, delirium, paranoid ideation, and bizarre behavior.

Medical problems that cocaine worsens include pulmonary complications such as wheezing, exacerbation of asthma and fluid in the lungs, and heart complications such as chest pains, attacks, and enlarged hearts.

Add such physical problems as nervous system complications, headaches, kidney failure, and others, and it becomes obvious that this drug can have deleterious effects on every organ in the human body. In one recent review article concerning cocaine abuse, some 50 complications were listed.

A complication deserving special mention is the adverse effect of this drug on an unborn child. The use of cocaine by a mother during pregnancy has been linked to lower infant birth weights, premature births, smaller heads, and neurobehavioral (nervous system and behavioral) dysfunction.

In addition to the direct toxicity of cocaine, it is associated with several other health problems. Sex sometimes is traded for drugs, resulting in increased risk for sexually transmitted diseases such as HIV/AIDS, gonorrhea, and syphilis.

Cocaine use has been connected with violent behavior

such as homicide and armed robbery. Studies have shown an increase in suicides and accidental deaths in users of this drug. It is not hard to see that cocaine use wreaks havoc in society by not only affecting individuals, but also their children, families, and communities.

The indirect complications also should be noted. Everyone is affected in some way by cocaine use, even if one is not a personal user nor acquainted with one.

The impact financially in costs to the community affects everyone. Every member of society is at risk for adverse outcomes from the use of this drug, including the spread of HIV/AIDS.

Marijuana: Many experts feel drug use among young people develops in predictable stages consistent with what is called "the gateway concept." This concept is that experimentation with drugs usually begins with cigarettes, alcohol, or marijuana, and then progresses to other "hard" drugs.

Use of marijuana prior to age fifteen has been associated with both heavier use after fifteen and the progression to the use of other drugs. The direct medical consequences of marijuana are not as well documented as those we see in cocaine users, but there are serious pulmonary (lung) consequences in heavy long-term users.

The evidence that marijuana can lead to the use of other drugs in adolescents should be taken very seriously. Of particular concern is the high rate of drug usage found among school dropouts and lower income, inner-city youth. The rates of drug use among these groups have increased more than the rates among the general youth population.

Conclusion

Illicit drug use poses serious consequences for users and society at large. Programs such as "Just Say No" that

address primary prevention and effective rehabilitation programs should be widely supported.

Political representatives and health policy members
must be made to understand that development and financial support of such programs is a societal mandate.

Every one of us must do his or her part if we are ever to
rid our communities of this ill which has such far-reaching,
devastating consequences.

Alcohol Abuse

by A. Maria Newsome, M.D.

A large percentage of Americans drink alcohol, and while modest amounts often result in few, if any, problems for many individuals, millions of others drink to the point of harm, both physical and emotional.

Contrary to popular opinion, most alcoholics are not "skid-row bums" but members of the work force or housewives.

Alcohol can have adverse effects on virtually every part of the body. For example, chronic and heavy alcohol consumption may lead to an enlarged heart, heart failure, an abnormal heart rhythm, or elevated blood pressure. Also, there is a connection between strokes and alcoholism, usually within twenty-four hours of drinking heavily.

These complications are quite prevalent. In fact, diseases of the heart and blood vessels are the leading cause of death in alcoholics. Cancer is the second most frequent cause of death in alcoholics. Certain sites in the body of an alcoholic may be up to ten times more likely to develop cancer than the same locations in non-alcoholics.

The most frequent cancers in alcoholics include head and neck cancer and cancer of the esophagus, stomach, liver, pancreas, and breasts.

The gastrointestinal tract is another area hit particularly hard by excessive alcohol intake, because alcohol causes inflammation of the esophagus and stomach. This may result in internal bleeding, stomach pain, and a poor appetite. It may also interfere with the absorption of nutrients, including B vitamins.

Excessive alcohol intake also is a very common cause of pancreatitis (inflammation of the pancreas) that frequently manifests as severe knifelike pain in the stomach area that radiates through to the back, as well as nausea and vomiting.

Although most cases of acute pancreatitis can be resolved with conservative measures, each episode is potentially life threatening. If a person continues to drink, the episodes of acute pancreatitis can progress to chronic pancreatitis, in which continuous or intermittent pain is so severe that it is difficult to control.

Also, since the pancreas makes insulin, damage from alcohol may result in diabetes. Malnutrition is a possibility, because the pancreas also makes essential proteins crucial to the body's ability to absorb nutrients.

One symptom of malnutrition, which people may not notice quickly, is a greasy texture to his or her stools due to the inability to absorb fat appropriately.

The Liver Is Very Susceptible to Alcohol Damage

Another organ targeted by alcohol is the liver. In fact, there is an entire spectrum of liver disease due to alcohol, including *fatty liver, inflammation of the liver called hepatitis,* and *cirrhosis* of the liver.

With a fatty liver, there is an accumulation of fat that enlarges the liver, but the person may have no symptoms. Or he may experience pain and tenderness in the upper abdomen below the right rib cage at the site of the liver. *If* a person who has developed this condition will stop drinking, these changes reverse, and the liver again becomes healthy.

If he or she continues to drink, the next potential problem is inflammation of the liver, called *hepatitis*. This generic term covers inflammation caused by other agents, such as viruses, as well. This condition also is potentially reversible. However, hepatitis *can* be life threatening.

There may be no symptoms, but there may be nausea, vomiting, and abdominal pain. Other signs include yellowing of the skin and the whites of the eyes, called *jaundice*, fever, poor appetite, and weight loss. Our grandparents' generation used to call this "yellow janders (jaundice)."

Cirrhosis is the final stage of liver damage. With cirrhosis, the liver is permanently scarred. It takes a number of years of excessive alcohol intake to develop this condition. However, the term *excessive* is relative.

Different bodies have different thresholds of alcohol intake above which severe liver damage is caused. Even what someone considers "moderate" drinking, if continued over an extended period of time, can result in cirrhosis.

Women in general have a lower threshold for alcohol-related liver disease than men, due to a difference in body chemistry.

A woman who drinks the equivalent of two or three beers a day for an extended period of time may have more bodily damage than a man who drinks the equivalent of four or five beers a day over the same period.

(One beer has about the same alcohol content as one and a half ounces of whiskey or four ounces of wine.)

With cirrhosis, a person may be symptom-free, or he may experience jaundice, anemia, shrunken testicles in males, enlarged breasts in males, menstrual irregularities in women, easy bruising, or fluid accumulation in the abdominal cavity resembling pregnancy, called *ascites* (a-sight-ees).

A very serious and potentially fatal complication of cirrhosis is the enlargement of blood vessels, called *varices* (ver-i-cees), in the esophagus which may rupture. If they do rupture, there is the potential of bleeding to death. Vomiting massive quantities of blood is the most common symptom of ruptured esophageal varices.

Most patients with advanced cirrhosis die in a coma induced by liver failure itself. The long-term outlook for this condition is poor. Less than half of those who have had a major complication of cirrhosis *and continue to drink* will be alive five years later.[1]

Other Areas That Alcohol Affects

The nervous system is yet another major part of the body affected by excessive alcohol intake. Nerve damage may manifest as burning, numbness, or tingling in the hands and feet, as well as other problems.

The brain itself may actually shrink over time in those who drink heavily.

Alcohol also can result in a number of adverse mental and psychological influences, some of which can be irreversible.

Alcohol abuse frequently leads to potentially serious nutritional deficiencies that, as an indirect cause of alcohol, may affect many parts of the body adversely. This is particularly true in pregnant women, in which case the unborn baby may be damaged.

In *fetal alcohol syndrome*, the baby may have a small head, mental retardation, heart defects, little teeth, an abnormal face, and other defects, as well as be born addicted also to alcohol. There is no set limit of alcohol intake above which this syndrome consistently occurs; therefore, it is recommended that all pregnant women completely stop drinking during pregnancy.

Alcohol abuse not only has the potential of destroying the mind and body, it often destroys other aspects of a person's life before that final stage is reached. Many potential alcoholics refuse to believe they have a problem. Their image of alcoholics is the "town drunk," or homeless bums lying passed out in the street somewhere.

However, the overwhelming majority of alcoholics do not fit this profile, as mentioned earlier.

Many physicians use a certain series of questions, called the CAGE *Questions*, as a screening test for alcohol abuse in their patients:[2]

Have you ever felt the need to Cut down on drinking?

Have you ever felt Annoyed by criticism of drinking?

Have you ever had Guilty feelings about drinking?

Have you ever taken a morning "Eye opener"?

The more "yes" answers a person has to these questions, the higher the likelihood that he or she has a drinking problem. It is important to know that alcohol abuse does not just manifest in someone drinking to the point of passing out, or even indulging to the point of drunkenness.

Alcohol abuse can be much more subtle. Many of those who consider themselves "social drinkers" actually are alcoholics.

Encouraging a loved one or friend to "cut back," or resolving to cut back yourself, will give you a good picture of whether or not you or they are addicted. Some people can cut back on their own, but others need a tremendous amount of support from family and friends, as well as support groups, including physicians.

It is natural to try to get a loved one to go "cold turkey," but there are some facts to keep in mind in this case. The most obvious and important one is that, if a person has been drinking excessively for a long time (even social drinking), various uncomfortable and potentially dangerous conditions may develop if he or she abruptly leaves off a substance to which the body has become accustomed, namely alcohol.

Withdrawal Symptoms Range From Mild to Serious

Usually, withdrawal symptoms are of mild medical significance although they may be very uncomfortable for the patient.

For example, less than ten hours after decreasing alcohol intake, a hand tremor, difficulty in sleeping and bad dreams, anxiety, stomach upset, and elevated temperature, pulse, or respiratory rates may develop. These symptoms may be most intense on day two or three but usually improve by day four or five, although some of them might persist for several months.

Approximately 5 percent of alcoholics experience severe withdrawal symptoms including confusion and/or hallucinations of sight, sound, or touch. A small percentage experience one or two seizures within forty-eight hours of abstinence from alcohol.

Although the majority of withdrawal syndromes are mild or self-limiting, some people experience a severe form of withdrawal that is potentially deadly. This is called *delirium tremens*, commonly known as "the DTs."

People experiencing this syndrome have considerable tremors to the point of shaking the entire body as in a severe chill and literally become delirious. Jokes about "pink elephants" may sound funny, but in reality, are anything but! Often people experiencing this severe a withdrawal also will develop fevers, fast heart rates, and major bouts of sweating.

In fact, delirium tremens is considered a medical emergency, because it has the potential to be fatal. It usually occurs between two and four days after a heavy drinker stops his or her alcohol intake. Therefore, if a person develops shaky hands twelve hours after his last drink, it is not considered DTs. Anyone with potentially severe withdrawal symptoms should be seen by a physician as soon as possible or taken to an emergency room.

The possibility of experiencing severe withdrawal symptoms should not be used as an excuse to continue drinking, for the number of people who die each year of DTs pales in comparison to the number that die from complications of chronic alcohol abuse.

The important thing about withdrawal is knowing when mild symptoms are progressing to the potentially dangerous stage and seeking medical attention early. *In most cases*, there may be physically and psychologically uncomfortable symptoms, but they will not become medically serious.

For those so inclined, instead of going "cold turkey," a person may want to consider cutting back gradually on alcohol consumption over a period of time. In this case, the chronic abuser should set a goal of a certain period of weeks to months — not years — in which to be completely off alcohol.

The ramifications of long-term alcohol abuse are tremendous, both in terms of physical and psychological suffering with respect to years of life lost, figuratively and literally.

Acknowledging that one has a problem is the first step in healing, and it is never too late to quit! Feelings of guilt and shame frequently make withdrawing harder and are counterproductive to letting go of the crutch of alcohol.

Everyone has weaknesses of various kinds. True strength comes in admitting those shortcomings and working toward overcoming them, rather than being overcome by them.

[1]Isselbacher K., et al; *Harrison's Principles of Internal Medicine*, 13th Ed. (New York: McGraw-Hill, Inc., 1994).

[2]Mayfield, D, McLeod, G., Hall P., *American Journal of Psychiatry*, "The CAGE Questionnaire," 1974; 131: p. 1121.

Cigarette Smoking
by A. Maria Newsome, M.D.

The number one *preventable* cause of death in America is cigarette smoking. It is believed to be responsible for close to 400,000 premature deaths each year. In other words, one out of every six deaths in the United States can be traced in some way to cigarette smoking.

Also, smokers are much more likely to be disabled due to chronic illnesses and more likely to miss days of work than non-smokers.

More than 4,000 substances have been identified in cigarette smoke, some of which cause cancer, and others that have different adverse effects on the body. Various factors are involved in these early deaths due to cigarette smoking, such as:

- The number of cigarettes smoked
- The number of years the person has smoked
- The depth of inhalation
- The strength of the cigarettes smoke

Hardly anyone today is not aware of the connection between smoking and lung cancer, but most people do not realize the many other potentially lethal conditions also associated with smoking tobacco.

As we have mentioned in earlier sections, an estimated 100,000 heart-attack deaths every year are attributed to smoking. Also, cigarette smoking, high LDL cholesterol, and hypertension are the three main risk factors for coronary artery disease.

If someone has two of these risk factors, he has approximately four times the risk of someone without them. And, if he has all three, there is eight times the risk.

Sudden heart-related deaths are more likely to occur in young male smokers than in non-smokers. Women who smoke and use birth control pills are about ten times more likely to develop coronary artery disease than women who use neither.

After a heart attack, those who continue to smoke are more likely to die of complications than those who quit. Also, cigarette smoking may interfere with the effectiveness of medication used to treat heart disease.

Also as mentioned in an earlier article, cigarette smoking is a contributing factor to strokes. Approximately 27,000 deaths a year from strokes are believed to be due to smoking.

Although smoking is not a risk factor for high blood pressure per se, hypertensive patients who do smoke have a greater chance of developing potentially catastrophic hypertension and dying from complications.

Smoking is the single most important cause of cancer deaths in this country, being responsible for close to 30 percent of these deaths with the number one cause of cancer deaths being lung cancer.

It has been estimated that those who smoke one pack a day increase their risk of developing lung cancer ten times over that of those who do not smoke. Those who use two packs a day increase their risk factors twenty-five times.

Other forms of cancer related to cigarette smoking (and/or chewing tobacco and dipping snuff) include cancers of the mouth and throat, bladder, pancreas, esophagus, kidney, stomach, cervix in women, and certain blood cells (myelocytic leukemia).

Aside from the potential for fatal diseases, cigarette smoking can cause major day-to-day suffering from chronic breathlessness and other symptoms, preventing the smoker from full enjoyment of daily life.

We discussed chronic obstructive pulmonary (lung) disease earlier, as well. This consists of emphysema and chronic bronchitis and kills tens of thousands each year.

The major culprit once again is tobacco. Men who smoke may have up to twenty-five times the likelihood of dying from lung problems as men who do not smoke.

Smokers are more apt to have respiratory infections.

Smokers are more likely to die from flu and pneumonia than non-smokers.

Smokers also are more likely to suffer respiratory complications after surgery than non-smokers, even when the surgery has nothing to do with smoking-caused problems.

Certainly, pregnancy and smoking do not mix, any more than pregnancy and alcohol consumption do. Infants born to mothers who smoked during pregnancy are more likely to weigh less.

Their mothers' smoking habits also may have negative effects on the infants' growth and intellectual development as compared to those infants whose mothers did not smoke. Finally, babies of smoking mothers are more likely to die before and after delivery.

Ulcers are more common in smokers than non-smokers, and in some cases, much more severe. Even second-hand smoke has been shown to cause cancer, respiratory problems, and heart disease in innocent, non-smoking bystanders.

Many smokers feel that they have indulged in this habit so long, there is no point in trying to quit because "the damage already has been done." *However, this is not true!* It is true that much damage caused by smoking cannot be reversed, but when a person stops smoking, the overall health status improves almost immediately.

A year after quitting, a person has a substantially decreased risk of suffering a heart attack. As a whole, it is a proven fact that former smokers tend to live longer than those who never stop smoking.

A second reason most smokers, particularly women, give for not quitting is that they will gain weight. True, they *may* gain a few pounds, but the slight potential for mild adverse effects due to the average amount of weight gained when a person stops smoking is in no way comparable to the tremendous health benefits that person will receive.

As far as appearance goes, it would be better to live a quality life a little overweight than to live a low-quality life with the potential of an early death, would it not?

It is always possible to deal with weight gain through exercise and diet, which in turn, would also add to the quality of life.

Most ex-smokers quit on their own, with many of them going "cold turkey." However, for those who have a great deal of difficulty kicking the habit, there are a variety of aids available, such as: group counseling, nicotine patches or gum prescribed by a physician, and so forth.

The nicotine replacement therapy should only be done under a physician's care, because it can be dangerous for certain people and there are special instructions concerning its use.[1]

Although many people experience unpleasant withdrawal symptoms when they attempt to give up nicotine, such as anxiety and difficulty concentrating, these symptoms are short-lived. However, the potential devastation of a heart attack, stroke, or any of the other major complications of smoking may last a lifetime — a needlessly shortened lifetime.

It is not too late to stop. If you are a smoker reading this, then today is a particularly good day to stop when all of this information is fresh in your mind.

Do not be discouraged if you do not make it on the first try. Many people have to try several times before they can completely get free of this highly addictive substance. You will never lose if you keep trying until you succeed!

[1]Isselbacher, K., et. al. *Harrison's Principles of Internal Medicine,* 13th Ed. (New York: McGraw-Hill, Inc., 1994).

Obesity

by A. Maria Newsome, M.D.

Obesity is a very common condition that often causes not only significant psychological difficulties, but carries significant medical risks as well. Although there are a few medical conditions that may contribute to obesity, most cases have no disease origin.

Obesity is more common in the black community as well as in other low socioeconomic groups, partly due to economic conditions and partly due to lack of education concerning good nutrition. There also is a lack of knowledge about what obesity can do to harm the body.

Aside from fruits, vegetables, and grains, some low-calorie items cost more than their high-calorie counterparts, such as a three-pound loaf of lean turkey meat versus three pounds of fat-laden pork. However, it is much better to spend more money on groceries and less on medical bills than to skimp on groceries and risk an early grave.

Obesity is associated with a significantly increased risk of the following medical problems:

Hypertension, heart attacks, strokes, diabetes, certain types of cancer, potentially serious breathing problems, gallstones, osteoarthritis, low back pain, as well as others.

Another problem contributing to obesity is that many people first become overweight during childhood and the habit of overeating and under-exercising sometimes is as difficult to break as that of smoking.

Therefore, it is extremely important for parents to begin instilling good eating habits in their children at an early age to try to curtail health problems later in life.

People have different metabolic rates, so that some can eat whatever they want and remain slim or even "skinny," while others eat relatively little and remain overweight. Recently, researchers have found that there may be a significant hereditary component to some individuals' propensity to be thin or overweight. However, this theory ought not to be used as an excuse to overlook other factors in obesity.

Even some people whose parents are overweight may not be overweight themselves because of a hereditary factor. Their own obesity may be attributed to habits of overeating developed in childhood and to living a non-active lifestyle.

The parents may have been overweight for these same reasons, so that the phrase "obesity runs in the family" often is more a matter of environmental learned behavior than of any genetic component.

However, there *are* those people who exercise regularly, watch what they eat, but still have difficulty getting down to an ideal body weight. Most of these people tend to finally give up on trying to control their weight.

For these people, in spite of perhaps not having much success in losing weight, it is important to keep exercising and watching their diets. The reason is to keep from gaining even more weight, thus putting them at an even greater risk of medical complications from obesity.

The important thing is to be checked out by a doctor and explore the most likely causes for being obese in your particular case. You can even find out for yourself by beginning a moderate exercise program and going on a reasonable diet. If you do not begin to lose weight within a reasonable time — say a month — then go to a doctor for help.

When a person attempts to lose weight, he should set realistic goals and not try to lose a great deal of weight in a short period of time. Not only will the weight be gained back easily, the person may become ill.

The key to successful, lasting weight loss is to *modify one's lifestyle.* Just as with persons wanting to avoid certain diseases or conditions or to improve their life spans after recovering from a serious disease, anyone wanting to lose weight should *learn to read labels on food packages.*

By carefully reading labels and through comparison shopping, an astute consumer can decrease the total number of calories he consumes to a significant extent. This person can maintain a nutritious, healthy diet at the same time.

Regular exercise is of vital importance in losing and keeping off weight. Those who exercise regularly have a higher life expectancy on an average than those who lead inactive lifestyles. Furthermore, an article in a recent issue of the *New England Journal of Medicine* shows a significant association between obesity and a decreased life expectancy.

Obviously, obesity has the potential of causing a tremendous amount of suffering and of robbing a person of years of life. Different people lose weight best by different methods. No one method works for everyone.

The important thing is to *get started.* Make a decision to keep trying until you find the method or combination of diet and exercise that works best for you.

Glaucoma

by *William C. Hurd, M.D.: Ophthalmologist*

Glaucoma is about eight times more common in African-Americans than in Caucasians. It is an eye disease that gradually shrinks the visual field and:

1. Leads to blindness if left untreated.

2. Has practically no symptoms in its early stages.

3. Tends to "run in the family" and has a higher incidence after age forty.

4. Can be diagnosed by an ophthalmologist or optometrist, although I recommend an ophthalmologist for comprehensive medical or surgical glaucoma management.

The most common types of glaucoma do not cause pain. Therefore, sometimes people do not realize they have it.

The good news is, when it is treated in its early stages, loss of sight almost always can be prevented.

Most of the two to three million Americans who have glaucoma are able to maintain their lifestyles and stay active. By properly following the treatment plan outlined by a physician (ophthalmologist), glaucoma may be controlled and its obstacles overcome.

Glaucoma develops when there is excess fluid in the eyeball. Images and light create certain nerve signals, which are carried to the brain by the *optic nerve*. This nerve consists of many delicate fibers and is located toward the back of the eyeball. Fluid inside the eyeball is called *aqueous humor*.

Normally, this fluid drains out of the eye in about equal proportion to the amount produced. In glaucoma, too much fluid accumulates either because of abnormalities in the drainage system or because of impaired access to this system. This increased *intraocular pressure* of the fluid, aqueous humor, is believed to eventually damage the fragile optic nerve fibers.

One "trademark," or early symptom of glaucoma, is the slow, gradual loss of peripheral (side) vision. This usually is a sign that the optic nerve is being pushed in, or "cupped," due to pressure. If this intraocular pressure is not reduced, after an extended period of time, major vision loss can occur.

While there is no cure for this condition, millions of people with it have learned to manage successfully and to lead active lives in spite of it.

Many safe and effective medications are now available to help manage glaucoma and prevent it from worsening. Of these, many are in the form of eye drops, and it is important to know how to administer them properly.

Sometimes more than one kind are prescribed together. A patient should be diligent to ask questions of his physician in order to fully understand what is happening in his case.

If a person who develops glaucoma will follow his physician's advice, use the medication or medications as prescribed, and become as informed about his condition as possible, he will be very likely to overcome the challenges that accompany this condition.

Systemic Lupus Erythematosis (SLE)

by Benjamin F. Evans, M.D.: Internal Medicine

Systemic lupus erythematosis (SLE), also called simply *lupus*, is a disease of unknown cause that can affect virtually every organ system in the body. Originally, this disease was grouped in a category of disorders called "collagen vascular disorders," as it was mistakenly believed that it was due in large part to a primary abnormality in the supporting framework of blood vessels and other tissues which are partially made of a protein called *collagen*. It is now believed that the body is damaged by deposition of abnormal antibodies called *autoantibodies*, which the body incorrectly makes which destroy its own cells and tissues, both directly and indirectly.

It is the production of these autoantibodies with the inability of the body to reduce or suppress them that leads to many of the clinical manifestations of SLE.

The typical lupus patient is a female of child-bearing age, between twenty and forty years of age. The disease is more common in blacks, but it is also present in other races as well. The initial presentation may be very vague complaints of fever, fatigue, skin lesions, nausea, weight loss and joint pain. Clinical evaluation in this early stage may be normal, but as the disease progresses, autoantibodies and other criteria for SLE will be manifested.

Clinical manifestations of SLE may occur spontaneously or could be exacerbated by pregnancy, stress, infection, physical trauma or sunlight. The majority will most certainly have systemic (widespread) manifestations, such as fatigue, nausea, fever and weight loss. However, the most frequent symptoms involve the musculoskeletal system (muscles and bones) and manifest as swelling of the knuckles and next closest joints of the hands, the wrists and knees.

There may also be skin manifestations involving the hair, skin, or mucous membranes. These may be characterized by hair loss, sensitivity to light, blister-like lesions, or the classical malar (butterfly) rash which is a reddish rash over the cheeks and bridge of the nose.

More serious manifestations which could lead to suffering or death are kidney failure, seizures, brain hemorrhage, psychosis, imflammation of the heart valves and lining of the heart and heart failure. Infections may also increase mortality due to increased use of corticosteroids (a specific type of steroid) and immune-suppressing agents often used to treat this disease.

In order for the diagnosis of SLE to be valid, four of the following eleven criteria should be evidenced at some time:

1. Butterfly rash (malar rash).

2. Discoid lupus (a specific skin rash).

3. Photosensitivity (sensitivity of the skin to light).

4. Oral ulcers.

5. Arthritis.

6. Inflammation of the lining of certain body organs.

7. Kidney disorders, seizures and psychosis.

8. Neurological disorders, such as seizures and psychosis.

9. Blood disorders, such as low white blood cells, red blood cells, or platelets.

10. Immune system disorders characterized by the presence of antibodies made against the body's own DNA or other specific components.

11. Antibody directed against the nucleus of cells.

Some drugs, such as certain oral contraceptives and a few of the drugs used to treat tuberculosis, hypertension and abnormal heart rhythms, can cause a "lupus-like" syndrome. The most common manifestations are fatigue, malaise (generally feeling bad), weight loss, nausea, fever and arthritis of multiple joints, but there are usually no brain or kidney disorders. Drug-induced lupus is usually distinguished from classic lupus by the presence of a specific class of antibodies.

Treatment of SLE should be based on severity of the disease. For mild disease due to stress, simple bed rest may be all that is needed. Typically corticosteroids, anti-inflammatory drugs that are not steroids, such as ibuprofen, salicylates (aspirin products) and even some drugs primarily used to treat malaria may be used for skin and musculoskeletal disorders. For moderate disease, such as inflammation of the lining of the lungs or heart, corticosteroid pills are used, and for severe disease, such as kidney involvement, brain inflammation and lung hemorrhage (bleeding), high doses of steroids, with or without other medications, are used.

It should be noted that there is no cure for SLE, and treatment should be directed toward acute flare-ups and maintenance. Because of improved treatment, the survival of SLE patients is better today and many patients are living longer. But the disease is usually characterized by symptom-free periods with intermittent periods when the disease can vary from mild to severe. Patients with severe involvement of the kidneys, brain, heart and lungs will usually have more suffering as well as a higher death rate.

Cancer and Abnormal Growths

.

Prostate and Colorectal Cancer

by A. Maria Newsome, M.D.

Prostate cancer is the *most common cancer* in American men, although lung cancer is the most common cause of cancer-related death. For reasons not fully understood, prostate cancer is more common and often more aggressive in blacks than in whites.

The American Cancer Society recommends that men aged fifty and over have a yearly digital rectal exam and a Prostate Specific Antigen (PSA) blood test. This antigen is often elevated in prostate cancer, although there can be other reasons for its elevation.

Also, prostate cancer is found when autopsies are done on many elderly men who died from causes completely unrelated to the cancer. This is because it sometimes takes decades for symptoms to occur in prostate cancer.

Because this cancer is often more aggressive in blacks, some have recommended screening for it at an earlier age than in the population at large. However, at present, the American Cancer Society has not recommended any special guidelines for black males, although it would be good for African-American males to be aware of this potential threat to their health.

Symptoms that *could* be related to prostate cancer include pain or discomfort in urination, difficulty in urinating (specifically in initiating the urine flow), pain in the back or hip, blood in the urine, or blockage of urine flow (due to growth of the cancer). If any man experiences any of these symptoms, particularly if he is over forty, he should seek medical attention.

However, you need to realize that there are other potential causes for these symptoms. For example, in the majority of cases of back pain in a forty-year-old male (or older), this has nothing to do with prostate cancer. However, any of these symptoms may stem from something else that needs to be treated.

Colorectal Cancer

Each year in this country, tens of thousands of people die from colorectal (colon/rectal) cancer. The good news is that this kind of cancer has a very high cure rate when caught early.

Common factors that increase the risk of developing colorectal cancer include a high-fat, low-fiber diet, advancing age, and a first-degree relative who has had this same type of cancer. (First-degree relatives include parents, siblings, and children.)

Preventive medicine is very important in today's health care. Instead of waiting to treat an advanced, often incurable, disease, doctors and patients alike are moving more toward preventive or early-care management measures. Because of this, potentially fatal diseases are often caught when they are still curable.

In the early stages, many diseases have no symptoms, so the old philosophy of only seeing a doctor when you are very sick should be discarded. Regular doctor checkups and visits can result in life-saving early diagnosis and intervention.

For those who do seek comprehensive medical care as

a preventive measure, the World Health Organization (WHO) recommends the following guidelines:

1. Have a digital ("digit" meaning the examiner's finger) examination each year beginning at age forty.

2. Have a fecal (referring to feces, or stool) occult (hidden or not readily visible to the eye) blood test each year beginning at age fifty. (This test is done from a sample of a stool taken from the physician's glove after he has done a digital rectal exam.)

3. A sigmoidoscopy done every three to five years beginning at age fifty. (This involves inserting a narrow instrument into the rectum by which a physician can look for signs of colon cancer.)

The sigmoidoscopy is something people used to dread. However, now it can be done in a doctor's office and requires no sedatives.

The newer flexible instruments are more comfortable than the old, rigid ones. There still is a mild to moderate amount of discomfort involved, but nothing like that involved in the old procedure. It takes only a few minutes and can literally affect the years one lives by helping diagnose colon cancer early.

Signs and symptoms of colorectal cancer vary, depending on a number of factors, such as the location of the cancer. Some symptoms include a change in bowel habits, rectal bleeding, or rectal pain.

For example, if a man or woman over fifty has always had one well-formed bowel movement a day but now has consistent diarrhea or constipation, he or she should seek medical attention.

Of course, these symptoms may also have other causes. Even if you experience one or more of these, do not assume that you have cancer. Just go and be examined in order to know for sure.

Many cases of this kind of cancer have no symptoms until the cancer is well-advanced. Colorectal cancer, like many other diseases, does not have to continue to claim so many lives. Appropriate preventive measures can save many people who otherwise would have died from this potentially fatal disease.

Even if your insurance does not pay for a sigmoidoscopy, this procedure is usually less than $200, so save up for it. This only needs to be done every three to five years, and it can literally save your life!

An "ounce of prevention" when it comes to your health certainly is worth much more than "a pound of cure" that may be too late.

Cervical Cancer

by Yvette Randle, M.D.: Family Practice

Screening for disease is an integral part of preventive medicine and has long been associated with routine office gynecologic examinations. However, cancer of the cervix is the only cancer for which there has been long-term and widespread screenings.

The incidence of this type of cancer is 13 per 100,000 women. There has been a dramatic reduction in the occurrence of invasive cancer because preinvasive cancerous changes can be recognized by a test known as the PAP (Papanicolaou) smear. This test is relatively inexpensive, painless, and accurate.

The frequency with which this smear needs to be taken is still being debated, with recommendations from various authorities ranging from every one to three years. However, the generally accepted guideline is once a year for single, sexually active females. More frequent tests would be advisable for those with a history of abnormal test results.

High-risk factors for cervical cancer include having multiple sexual partners, beginning sexual intercourse at an early age, and having several children. Recent evidence has shown that the presence in the body of certain subtypes of the virus that causes genital warts (human papillomavirus) significantly increases the risk of cervical cancer.

This virus is sexually transmitted, which probably accounts for the fact that women who have had multiple sex partners are at a much higher risk than women who have had only one partner. Another risk factor is the use of nicotine.

The average age of those developing cervical cancer is decreasing from the mid-fifties a few decades ago to the forties today. It is as yet seldom seen before age twenty.

Studies from the National Cancer Institute (NCI) suggest, however, that the younger the patient, the more aggressive the cancer. NCI studies list this as the most common invasive cancer in women ages twenty-five to twenty-nine and second most common among those aged thirty to thirty-four.[1]

There usually is no pain associated with this cancer until it is well advanced. Abnormal vaginal bleeding, especially after sexual intercourse, signals the need for a visit to one's physician as this *might* be a symptom. Vaginal bleeding outside of menses warrants evaluation by a physician.

Cases with no symptoms can still be detected by having regular PAP smears. Fortunately, cervical cancer grows relatively slowly and, if detected in time, is curable.

[1]Mishell, M.R., Bremmer, P. R., *Obstetrics and Gynecology*, (M.A. Blackwell Scientific Publications, 1994), 3rd. Ed.

Uterine Fibroids

by Yvonne Sims, M.D.:
Obstetrics and Gynecology

Uterine fibroids are the most common abnormal growths in a female pelvis and are benign (non-cancerous) tumors of the uterine muscle. Between 30 and 50 percent of black women over the age of thirty-five are estimated to have uterine fibroids.

The size, shape, and location of fibroids vary greatly, with some being very small and causing no problems and others becoming large enough to fill the pelvis and be mistaken for pregnancy.

Also, it is not clear exactly what causes them; however, once they do occur, their growth seems to be influenced by the hormone estrogen.

This explains why they often grow larger during pregnancy or when a woman is taking oral contraceptive pills with a high dosage of estrogen. During menopause, when estrogen levels fall, fibroids tend to become smaller and often disappear.

Treatment for fibroids must of necessity be individualized because of the variances in them. If the fibroids are small and causing no symptoms and if the patient is near or after menopause, usually there is no treatment at all. However, the patient should be checked regularly by a physician for any changes.

There *are* some signs or symptoms that may signal the need for treatment. These include:

• Progressively heavy, lengthy, and/or painful menstrual cycles, particularly when accompanied by anemia.

• Bleeding between periods.

• A suspicion that the growth might be an ovarian tumor rather than a fibroid.

• It becomes large enough to obstruct the urinary system.

• Rapid growth that might indicate an extremely rare development of a malignancy.

When treatment does become necessary, a hysterectomy is not always the treatment of choice. Depending on the woman's age and child-bearing desires, other treatment methods can and should be considered. No single approach to this problem will be right for every woman.

A patient should discuss all treatment options with her physician, and then together, they should select a plan that fits her particular needs.

Breast Cancer and Breast Self-Examination

by Melrose Blackett, M.D.:
Obstetrics and Gynecology

Everyone has the primary responsibility for his or her own health. This is particularly true for women in the area of their breasts. A doctor can only do his part if you do yours.

Performing a monthly breast self-examination (BSE) is a very important part of this responsibility because it is the best way to detect breast cancer in its early stages.

Why examine your own breasts?

Self-examination has been shown to be the best defense a woman has against breast cancer. Approximately 182,000 women were diagnosed with breast cancer in 1994, and American Cancer Society statistics show that one in nine American women will develop breast cancer at some time in their lives.

This does not have to be as frightening as it sounds. If detected early, this kind of cancer can be treated with good results. The following facts will bear this out:

• Most breast lumps are not found by doctors, but by the women themselves, either by accident or during a self-examination.

• Most breast lumps (more than 80 percent of them) are benign (non-cancerous) and, therefore, not life-threatening.

• Even if a lump is cancerous, the cancer can be cured in nine out of ten cases, if it is found early enough and if the cancer is confined to the breast.

• Early detection and prompt treatment have greatly increased the survival rate. The five-year survival rate for localized breast cancer has risen from 78 percent in the 1940s to 93 percent in 1994.

Breast self-examination is the key to early detection and can be life-saving. Every woman is at risk, as *breast cancer cannot be prevented!*

Research has shown that tumors found by women who practice BSE on a regular basis are half the size of tumors found by those who do not practice BSE. Smaller tumors have a greater chance to be contained within the breast if cancerous and, therefore, the patient has a much higher chance of survival.

When should a woman examine her breasts?

A woman should examine her breasts every month about a week after her menstrual cycle has ended. By waiting a week, any changes triggered by the cycle have had time to be resolved.

If a woman does not have monthly cycles due to being irregular, pregnant, having had a hysterectomy, or into or past menopause, she can just pick a certain date each month to do this exam. The point is to be consistent and regular.

What causes breast cancer?

In most cases, no one knows. An estimated 70 to 75 percent of women who develop breast cancers have no risk factors other than their age and being female! There *are* certain factors that have been linked to an increased risk, such as a personal or family history of breast cancer, the early onset of menstruation (before age thirteen), being over forty years of age, and of a higher educational and socioeconomic status — which is opposite to the risk factors of most diseases.

In addition, the NCI, the American Cancer Society, and the American Academy of Sciences have issued recommending guidelines on reducing fat intake to 30 percent in the average woman's diet, as well as reducing total fat intake.

A striking difference has been found between breast-cancer rates in countries where fat intake is higher compared to those where the diet is low in fat.

However, breast cancer is so common that every woman should be screened, a method of checking for disease when there are no symptoms.

What is a doctor's responsibility in this area?

Your doctor should include a thorough breast examination during your annual physical examination (which everyone should have). Any questions or concerns you may have should be addressed completely, and he should highlight the importance of BSEs.

He probably will recommend a mammogram, if you are over thirty-five years of age. After forty, one is recommended every two years, and after age fifty, every year.

How does a woman check for changes in her breasts?

Monthly breast exams enable a woman to become familiar with her own breasts and to gain confidence in her ability to perform BSEs. Many women fail to examine their breasts because they do not know how or are not sure how to do this.

The first thing to know is that normal breast tissue is composed of mainly fatty and glandular tissue and varies in consistency from woman to woman. The texture for each individual also varies at different times during the month.

Here are the steps in a BSE:

1. Stand in front of a large mirror and check both breasts for anything unusual — swelling, dimpling, bulges, skin changes, or changes in nipple texture.

2. Repeat this with your arms clasped behind your head.

3. Repeat with your hands firmly on your hips while contracting your chest muscles.

4. Examine both nipples for signs of spontaneous nipple discharge, also note color and consistency of any discharge when the nipples are *gently* squeezed.

5. Raise one arm and use the flat part of the fingers, not the fingertips, to feel for lumps or tender areas, which is easier to do while the breasts are wet and covered with soap or dry and powdered because of reduced friction.

Be sure to examine the entire breast using either lines, circles, or wedges, as seen in the diagram that follows. *Be sure to include the armpit area.*

6. Repeat #5 procedure while lying in bed with a pillow under one shoulder. This elevates and flattens the breast.

The keys to early breast cancer detection are:

Monthly breast self-examinations, annual breast examinations by a physician, and a mammogram when recommended. BSEs are not a substitute for mammograms or breast exams by a doctor.

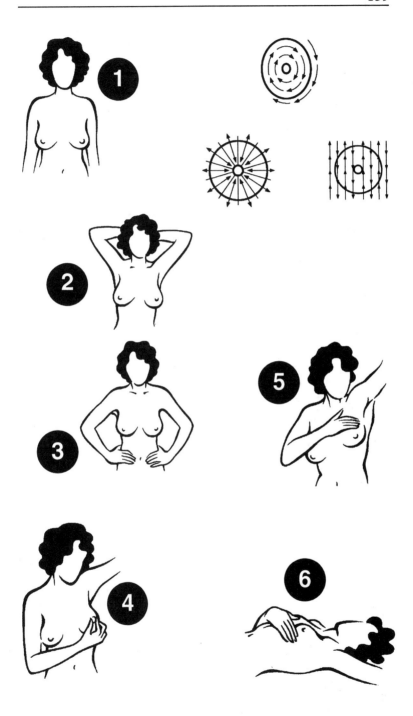

Sickle Cell Disease

by Loretta Bobo-Mosley, M.D.:
Internal Medicine

Sickle cell disease is a hereditary disorder of the red blood cells' hemoglobin, the substance that binds oxygen in the cells, which is needed by all body tissues. In the United States, this disease primarily affects African-Americans. The name comes from the appearance of the cell.

There are different genetic and clinical manifestations of this disease, so that medical care and lifestyle modifications cannot be planned on a general basis to fit everyone. The different expressions of this disease require different treatment.

People with this disease may look very healthy or appear chronically ill. Some must have frequent medical interventions, while others only need to be seen once or twice a year.

The disease is inherited and cannot be acquired.

Regardless of racial or ethnic origins, medical experts believe that all newborns should be screened to determine if the sickle cell gene is present.

In this country, the major forms of the disease are as follows:

Hemoglobin SS disease (sickle cell anemia), the severest form of the disease which affects about one in 400-625

African-Americans; Hemoglobin SC affecting approximately one in 833; and Hemoglobin S-beta thalassemia, affecting about one in 1,667 African-Americans. Hemoglobin S is the specific name used for sickle hemoglobin. Most persons have Hemoglobin AA. Other hemoglobins include C,D,E,F,H, and O.

However high the rate among African-Americans, the fact remains that Hemoglobin S disorders are the most common hemoglobin disorders in the world, affecting people of numerous ethnic origins.

Persons in Africa who live or whose ancestors lived in areas where malaria is or was prevalent may carry the sickle gene. In addition, the disease is found in Hispanics, Greeks, Turks, Italians, Arabs, Veddoid Indians, Cambodians, Vietnamese, and Laotians. Indeed, due to increasing racial admixture, the sickle gene may be found now in any ethnic group.

This disease is catastrophic, causing great physical and mental distress for those afflicted. It is associated with chronic suffering and early death.

A diagnosis can be made early in life either prenatally, neonatally, or postnatally. Universal screening of all newborns is indicated so that life preserving measures and parental education can be implemented while the child is at great risk.

The *sickle cell trait* (hemoglobin AS) is *not* included as part of the disease syndrome and should not be considered as sickle cell disease itself. Persons with the trait usually have less than 40 percent hemoglobin S and are therefore protected by the dominant normal hemoglobin A.

The trait affects about one in 12 African-Americans. Although there are problems associated with having the trait, it does not reach the same level of severity as the disease itself.

Some problems having high association with the trait

include possible damage to the spleen at altitudes of over 10,000, an inability to concentrate the urine, blood in the urine, bladder and kidney infections during pregnancies, and possible death from a type of malaria (caused by the organism Plasmodium Falciparum).

Other problems that may be associated with the trait include kidney and eye disease, death of certain bone tissue, and a rare occasion of sudden death associated with strenuous exercise (postulated as a cause in the deaths of some military recruits).

However serious all of those problems sound, the fact is that *the majority of persons with the sickle cell trait have no problems attributable to it.* Their life expectancies are the same as that of the general population's.

Characteristics of Sickle Cell Disease

Sickle cell disease, as differentiated from having the sickle cell trait, is characterized by chronic, intermittent, and painful episodes called "crises" and by a chronic hemolytic anemia (low red blood cell count due to a breaking open of the red blood cells). The chronic anemia tends to cause a decrease in exercise tolerance and easy fatiguability. When the red cells break down at a fast rate, the person's eyes may become yellow because of the hemoglobin breakdown.

Crises is a "catch phrase" used to describe the sudden onset of severe pain, with or without an associated fever. These crises are common in childhood as well as in adulthood and tend to be cyclical (to run in cycles). The pain syndrome may last hours to weeks with many possible precipitating factors, such as infections, fevers, dehydration, or sudden cooling.

Cells that have been subjected to repeated sickling become irreversibly "sickled." That means these cells can become trapped in small blood vessels, causing stasis, vasoocclusion (blockage of blood vessels), and regional ischemia (loss of blood and oxygen supply). A vicious cycle of these conditions results in tissue destruction and, ultimately, organ failure.

Infants are protected from these crises by high levels of fetal hemoglobin (hemoglobin F) up to the first three to six months of life. Hand or foot pain and swelling is the most common form of crisis for children under age five. These children are also at great risk for life-threatening meningitis (infection of brain tissue and lining) and generalized sepsis (infections).

Adults are more likely to complain of back, joint, and extremity pain that is not usually associated with significant swelling. Abdominal crises require careful examinations to rule out situations that might require surgery. No organ is spared.

Adults with sickle cell disease may suffer blindness, hearing loss, recurrent pneumonia, heart or kidney failure, joint pain and swelling, and leg ulcers. Females may have difficulty with conception and with carrying a baby to term. Males may suffer priapism (painful penile erections). Both children and adults are at risk for strokes, infections, and attacks of generalized pain.

The general types of treatment include identification and treatment of precipitating factors, usually infections such as sore throat, pneumonia or urinary tract infections, adequate hydration (fluids), and pain medication and therapy. Measures to make the patient comfortable are very important. These measures include a quiet environment, the application of a warm blanket or heating pad, and reassurance. In general, the application of ice packs to swollen joints or febrile patients should be avoided.

Presently, all anemic sickle cell patients are recommended to take folic acid, but iron supplements are only indicated for those who have documented iron deficiencies.

Immunization with pneumococcal and influenza vaccines are recommended for all patients with this disease. The use of penicillin in prophylactic (preventive) doses has been shown to reduce the childhood incidence of pneumococcal sepsis (a life-threatening infection involving the blood stream) by 84 percent. Therefore, this therapy is presently being universally recommended for all *children* with sickle cell disease.

Some patients with sickle cell disease have been cured with allogeneic bone marrow transplants. For most, this is not a reasonable or economically feasible option. There are several drugs in clinical trials now that may soon result in major breakthroughs in therapeutic options for treating sickle cell disease.

These drugs include hydroxyurea and butyrate salts that increase the production of hemoglobin F (fetal hemoglobin). This type of hemoglobin, like hemoglobin A, decreases sickling and the untoward effects of hemoglobin S.

General counseling regarding diet, exercise, and travel must be individualized for every patient, many of whom require educating concerning specific psychological, socioeconomic, and genetic factors. Health maintenance and disease prevention methods also are of the utmost importance. This includes a minimum of an annual physical examination and age-specific health interventions, such as required or recommended vaccines, testicular exams, PAP smears, and mammograms.

Sickle cell disease not only has a devastating impact on the persons who are afflicted with it, but also on their families and caregivers. The disease also has a significant impact on the medical care facilities and industries in various communities, and all should be concerned that these individuals get the best possible medical care.

Preventive Dentistry

by Delois Roberson, DDS

An overview of physical health is incomplete without proper consideration of oral health. Regular dental exams are essential to good health. Some diseases — from chicken pox to AIDS — manifest oral signs and symptoms. You, your physician, and your dentist must work together to maintain your health.

You are the most important factor in maintaining your oral hygiene. A dentist cannot keep anyone's teeth healthy without that person's help. There are several things you can do to keep a healthy smile. Proper and daily home care are essential if your teeth are to last a lifetime.

Brushing and flossing will help reduce the number of bacteria that live in the mouth. Brushing not only reduces bacteria but stimulates blood supply to the tissues and aids in reducing the sugar and carbohydrates on which bacteria feed. Purchase an American Dental Association (ADA) approved toothpaste. Selecting the proper toothbrush is also very important. A toothbrush with soft bristles is recommended. Hard bristles tend to damage the tissue and teeth surfaces when used improperly.

The correct way to brush is to place the toothbrush at a 45-degree angle at the gum line. You should feel the bristles between the teeth and gums. Use a gentle, slow, circular motion. Brush all surfaces of the teeth and your tongue.

Brush for three to five minutes, two to three times a day. However, brushing alone is insufficient. The bristles of the brush will not remove all material effectively from between the teeth. Flossing allows the removal of food particles and other items that tend to become lodged between the teeth.

Flossing is most effective when the following steps are followed:

1. Wrap floss around your two index fingers, then brace the floss against your thumbs.

2. Slide the floss between the teeth.

3. Move it along the surfaces between the teeth and the gum line.

4. Use up-down strokes until surfaces are clean. Do not use a sawing motion; this will damage your tissue.

5. Be sure to keep the floss braced as you go down into the gum area.

6. Wrap the used portion around one index finger, and unwrap clean floss from the other finger.

7. Repeat these steps on each tooth.

Mouth rinses on the market have greatly improved in recent years. Rinses now contain properties that may reduce bacteria and aid in maintaining healthy gums. However, rinses do not remove tartar from your teeth. They will not prevent or cure oral disease. Research is still ongoing concerning their benefits and use in the control of gum disease.

Visit your dentist twice a year for an examination. Teeth are not the only concern of dentists. Actually, an examination begins when the patient enters the office. His or her gait (the way one walks) and general appearance can indicate signs of illness.

During the dental exam, an external examination of the face, fingers, glands, and temporomandibular (jaw) joints takes place. The internal exam includes more than the teeth. The surfaces of the lips, the cheeks, throat, glands, palate, floor of the mouth, tongue, and supportive structures of the teeth along with the teeth are checked for signs of disease.

Periodontal disease (sometimes referred to as gum disease or pyorrhea) continues to be the number-one cause of tooth loss over the age of thirty-five. It has been estimated by leading dental organizations that more than 80 percent of the United States population is affected by some form of gum disease. Tooth loss is *not* inevitable with age. Teeth can last a lifetime with proper oral health care and maintenance.

Periodontal disease is inflammation or infection of the gums and of the bone supporting your teeth. The primary cause is *plaque*, a hardened bacterial film that forms on the teeth. If not removed, the bacteria buildup will soon destroy the gums and the bone that supports your teeth. It is a painless disease that may progress rapidly.

There are many signs that may indicate periodontal disease, such as tender gums that may appear red, swollen, and bleed easily. The presence of pus, loose permanent teeth, and a persistent bad odor may indicate an advanced form of the disease.

Other factors that contribute to the risk, progression, and severity of periodontal disease include: food impacted between teeth, overhanging fillings, poorly fitting dental appliances, the use of tobacco, and malaligned teeth. Systemic diseases, such as AIDS or diabetes, poor eating habits, and some medications also may reduce the tissues' ability to ward off infection.

Adults must take the initiative to improve their children's and their own oral health.

Infants and Children: Parents can do several things that will help reduce decay in the teeth of their infants and children.

1. Do not let an infant keep its bottle while it sleeps. Allowing a child to sleep with a bottle in its mouth may result in rotten front teeth, called "baby bottle syndrome."

2. Keep children's tongues clean. An infant's tongue can be kept clean by wiping with a moist towel, and the same holds for the teeth when they begin to come in.

3. As soon as a child has several teeth, begin to help them brush the teeth and the tongue. Use a soft, small tooth-brush angled toward the gums and use a slow, circular motion over all tooth surfaces.

4. Do not allow baby teeth to decay or go untreated. A child will have some primary teeth until about age twelve. These teeth should be maintained because they will affect the position and development of the permanent teeth.

5. Look inside the child's mouth from time to time, and if you notice cavities or have questions, see a dentist.

The first dental visit should be scheduled when the child is two or three years of age. It is helpful to go over what will occur at the initial dental visit. Books and/or an actual scheduled pre-appointment visit will result in a pleasant first dental experience for your child.

An unpleasant first visit to the dentist may cause dental anxiety for life. Also, parents' attitudes toward taking care of their own teeth will greatly influence the value their children place on oral health care.

Adults' dental health is in their hands. The following tips will assist you as you move toward improving your oral health:

1. To ensure that you receive quality dental treatment, avoid only visiting your dentist on an emergency basis.

Quality care and learning about good dental health is the last thing on your mind in emergency cases. It is hard, if not impossible, to inform or educate someone in pain!

2. Avoid the "just-take-it-out" syndrome. Keep your teeth as long as you can, even if it means having a root canal done. Today, advances in techniques and materials have greatly decreased the discomfort experienced with root-canal therapy.

3. Teeth that have to be extracted should be replaced with the appliance recommended by the dentist as soon as possible to prevent the shifting of the remaining teeth.

4. Disease can be properly diagnosed and treated by professionals. You can expect to return to health sooner. Do not diagnose and treat yourself without professional help.

The **family** must take an active role in the prevention of dental disease. *Sealants*, substances a dentist can place on the teeth to prevent decay, are highly recommended for permanent teeth. Mouth guards will help minimize fractures of teeth and bone during athletic participation.

Prefabricated gold crowns are no longer fashionable as previously thought. Many individuals who had these placed years ago are now having them removed. Keep healthy, natural looking teeth. When a permanent tooth needs to be capped, a cast crown is recommended.

Establish a relationship with a dentist with whom you can feel comfortable. Visit twice a year or more if recommended. I am sure everyone basically would like to keep his or her own teeth for an entire lifetime. However, saving all your teeth may not be possible after years of neglect. It is greatly to your advantage to make a commitment to improve your oral health and that of your family's. Your dental health is in your own hands.

Allow the dentist to assist you in maintaining a healthy smile.

Prenatal Care

by Rhonda Sullivan-Ford, M.D.:
Obstetrics and Gynecology

The profile of the "typical" mother has changed dramatically within the last quarter century. There has been a significant increase in teen pregnancies on one end of the spectrum, while at the other, many women are waiting until they are in their thirties and forties before having children.

Nevertheless, following is a brief overview of some important information all new mothers should have.

In spite of the many sophisticated technological neonatal intensive care units across the country and the excellent prenatal care that is now available, the infant mortality rate is not as low as should be expected. In fact, the mortality rate has increased over the past five years.

For this reason, it is important to try to plan your pregnancy. Some of the benefits include a chance to stop cigarette smoking, alcohol use, and drug abuse. Also, if a pregnancy is planned, nutrition supplementation with folic acid can decrease the chance of birth defects. Glucose control for diabetes can be implemented early.

Any woman who becomes pregnant should seek prenatal care early and find out what she can do personally to make the next few months safer for herself and her baby.

Every woman should keep a calendar on which she records the days of her monthly menstrual cycle. This is a good place to note any unusual events (heavy discharge, unusual pains) that may occur in that month.

One of the first questions asked by a physician or nurse during the first prenatal visit is, "When was the first day of your last menstrual period?"

This information is compared with the size of the baby on physical exam or ultrasound and is used to determine the due date. The more accurate this information, the better your health care providers can serve you. If the patient can provide this information readily, it will assist the health care worker in devising a treatment plan.

Also, it is important for everyone to know her medical history. For example, women with high blood pressure, sickle cell disease, diabetes, or systemic lupus erythematosus are considered "high risk." Actually, women with these diseases should consult a physician *before* becoming pregnant.

Complications accompanying these diseases which can arise during pregnancy are beyond the scope of this overview; however, a woman can discuss these issues with her private physician.

A teenager who is unsure about her medical history or family medical history should try to obtain this information from her mother or other family member to take to the doctor on her first visit. Alternatively, she could have a family member accompany her on the initial prenatal visit to help answer pertinent questions. However, do not let not having this information delay your first visit. Your doctor will let you know if he or she needs more information.

A positive pregnancy test brings great responsibility, and one consideration of primary importance for a good outcome is good nutrition. It is very important to eat properly during pregnancy. Most women do not know the appropriate diet they need in pregnancy. Do not be afraid to ask questions about this. Small changes in diet and exercise are things under your control that can improve the outcome of your pregnancy.

A nutritionist can be very helpful in answering specific questions about diet, particularly for those women who start pregnancy underweight or overweight.

In addition to nutrition, there are three important *don'ts* for anyone who wants the best outcome for herself and her newborn baby:

1. Don't smoke. (Tobacco is a drug.)

2. Don't use alcohol.

3. Don't use street drugs.

Any woman who uses any of these substances should seek professional help to get off these potentially devastating chemicals. Not just the immediate, but the long-lasting, effects of drugs and alcohol on the baby and mother are phenomenal.

Following are some complications associated with use of tobacco, alcohol, and/or drugs: Preterm labor, low birth weight which also carries a risk of developing many diseases, death before and after labor (perinatal death), fetal alcohol syndrome, rupture of the placenta (*abruptio placenta*), fetal growth retardation, and potentially serious withdrawal symptoms for the baby which may be born addicted.

Most of these complications can be eliminated by ceasing to take the drug involved and getting good prenatal care. Some studies show that eliminating smoking during pregnancy could improve fetal well-being and decrease early infant deaths, i.e., Sudden Infant Death Syndrome (SIDS). Heart defects, limb defects, and bladder problems are only a few of the potential complications of cocaine abuse. The most serious effect is fetal demise, which occurs more frequently near term.

Consequences of Venereal Diseases

Another issue of utmost importance is screening pregnant women for sexually transmitted diseases. The American College of Obstetrics and Gynecology recommends screening for gonorrhea, chlamydia, syphilis, hepatitis, HIV, and other diseases.

The reason for this screening is not only for the benefit of the mother but for the benefit of the fetus. Sexually transmitted diseases can have a profound effect on an infant.

For example, mothers with syphilis can pass this disease on to the fetus. This can affect the baby's liver, spleen, teeth, eyes, and ears. In fact, infection from this disease can kill the fetus. All of this could be prevented with early diagnosis and treatment.

Gonorrhea and Chlamydia are two very common sexually transmitted diseases which can lead to preterm delivery or premature rupture of the membranes. If chlamydia is transmitted to the infant, an eye infection or even pneumonia may develop.

In addition to preventing these diseases from affecting one's child, women should insist condoms be used because both of the above diseases can cause pelvic inflammatory disease (PID). Of course, the use of condoms also aid in the prevention of pregnancy in the first place.

PID can leave such bad scar tissue around the reproductive organs that it can cause infertility. This scarring also significantly increases a woman's risk of having a tubal pregnancy. This can result in a woman's bleeding to death if not detected in time.

Infants born to mothers with hepatitis B will be vulnerable to this virus and may become "chronic carriers" of it. One in four of the infants born with this vulnerability is also susceptible to eventually developing cirrhosis or cancer of the liver. Treatment of the newborn, however, can reduce the chance of this life-threatening process ever developing.

Every pregnant woman ought to be offered a test for HIV, which can be transmitted to the infant before, during, or after the delivery. Such transmission cannot be prevented at this point, because the exact time when transmission takes place is not known. However, treating a woman during pregnancy and in labor and treating the baby for the first six weeks of life will decrease by 67 percent the chance that the baby contracts the infection.

Another sexually transmitted disease is *genital herpes*, although there is not much risk of transmitting this virus to the baby while it is in the womb. However, a woman with a history of this virus should tell her doctor because, if the virus is active at the time of delivery, the baby can be infected as it passes through the birth canal.

If this occurs, there is a high rate of mental retardation and even death. If a woman does have active herpes when it is time to deliver, the obstetrician will simply do a Caesarian (C-section), thus making it highly unlikely that the baby would suffer either of the consequences.

However, the doctor must be made aware of the infection in order to do a meticulous examination of the external and internal genitalia. He needs to look for potentially infectious secretions before allowing a baby to pass through the birth canal.

For the reasons discussed here and others, it is crucial for all pregnant women to contact a physician as soon as possible after they find out they are pregnant. Your health-care worker, medical doctor, and social worker can assist with many issues affecting health (i.e., smoking cessation, alcohol/drug abuse, nutritional problems, physical abuse, venereal disease). Please contact the above personnel for help with these important issues, preferably before pregnancy.

Routine prenatal care, nutrition, and early disease screening and treatment are of paramount importance in reversing the present trend of increased infant mortality in the African-American community.

Tips for Parenting

by Carolyn Whitney, M.D.: Pediatrics

Parenting is one of the most important — if not the most important — job anyone can have. It ought to be considered a career in itself. It can be stimulating, challenging, fulfilling, and yet frustrating, beyond compare.

The problem is that cute little infants who become toddlers, children, and then "raging" teenagers do not always read the child-care books! They do not seem to know how the books say they are supposed to act and grow.

Therefore, the only real hope one can have is prayer, patience, and common sense. Hopefully, the few pages of this article will help some weary "war-torn" parent through the maze of the process called *parenthood*.

Through the following tips concerning the multiple stages and phases of childhood, perhaps some will be helped.

Tips for newborns through older infants:

— Dress the infant appropriately. If it is warm outside, dress the baby to stay cool. If it is cold, put the infant into warmer apparel.

— Feed only breast milk or infant formula for the first several months. Checks with a doctor, clinic, or WIC office before adding foods such as cereal, fruits, vegetables, bread, meats, or juices.

— Early feeding does not prevent or stop colic. Introduction of infant foods is a developmental process.

Introducing baby foods too early may result in the development of food allergy.

— Most infants by the age of two or three months are sleeping ten to twelve hours at night in addition to naps during the day.

— A new mother would find it advisable to rest during the day whenever her baby takes a long nap.

— Holding the baby will not spoil him or her but builds rapport, security, and love.

— Immunizations begin at two months of age. During the first six months, the infant should receive three DPTs, three oral polio vaccines, three Type B influenza vaccines (hemophilus influenzae, Type B), and three hepatitis B vaccines.

— Formula should be continued until the infant is about a year old. The earliest age recommended to switch to homogenized milk is nine months, at which time, the American Academy of Pediatrics also recommends that iron-fortified vitamins be added. Too early introduction to cow's milk promotes anemia (iron-poor blood).

— The age for reaching developmental milestones are as individual as the different children. If a parent has any questions concerning a child's development, he or she should consult the pediatrician.

— A teaspoon means a measuring teaspoon, not the size teaspoon with which you eat. The same applies to a tablespoon.

— Temperature cannot be accurately gauged by touching a child's skin. When in doubt, take the child's temperature orally (by mouth), axillary (under the arm), or rectally (in the rectum). Rectal thermometers measure the actual body core temperature and are considered the most reliable instrument by which to determine fever.

— Infants and young children should be restrained in approved car seats. Children four years old and older, or weighing 40 pounds or more, should wear seat belts while traveling.

— Never turn your back on young children any more than you would with pit bulls and wild circus animals, not because they are dangerous to you, but because you have no idea what they will do next and how fast they can get away from you.

Falls from beds and changing tables, burns from pulled over cups or other containers of hot beverages or foods, drowning in just a few minutes in only a few inches of water can all happen faster than you could believe possible.

Many accidents can be prevented by using gates for open stairways, placing poisons and harmful cleaning products, etc. out of a child's reach, and fitting safety plugs over electric outlets.

— Propping up a bottle in the infant's mouth so he or she can be "pacified" at night and not wake up the parents is not worth it in light of the possible choking, ear infections, and early dental cavities that can result.

— Only use syrup of Ipecac as directed by the Poison Control Center. An old saying is very true, "If it's hot going down, it will be hot coming back up."

— Never put anything smaller than an elbow in the ear. That means that even cotton-tipped swabs push wax farther into the ear canal and defeat the purpose of cleaning.

Tips for the toddler and older child:

— Toilet training always should be based on the individual child, not necessarily on the age "Grandma" thinks or to keep up with a neighbor or relative. Probably it is best to attempt this between the ages of 18 and 24 months.

— *No* is the password for this age. A toddler often will say "no" even when he or she means "yes." This is a normal part of a toddler's learning that he is an individual in his own right.

— Visits to the dentist should begin as early as three years old, and good dental hygiene should begin long before that with the advent of the first tooth. Emphasis should be placed on keeping the teeth clean, and candies and sugar-laden sweets should be discouraged.

— Children at this age may have as many as six to seven colds a year.

— Controlling what your young child watches on television protects the mind and emotions the way you would the body.

— At this age, your child should have received five DPTs, four oral polio vaccines, two MMRs, one PPD, and five HIBs.

— Children up to age two are very prone to ear infections because of the fact that the ear canals have horizontal positioning. As the child grows older, positioning becomes more vertical as seen in the adult ear and infections should be less likely.

Tips for the adolescent:

— Good nutrition is still very important with a focus on calcium for strong bones, as well as on rich sources of iron.

— Menstruating females *must* examine their breasts monthly.

— Teenagers should receive three sets of hepatitis B vaccines, if he or she has not already had this series, and TD, and a second MMR.

— It is important to educate teenagers about sex and to keep the lines of communication open between parents and teens.

— Routine annual eye and dental exams are encouraged.

— Contrary to popular belief, chocolate, spicy foods, and carbonated beverages do not cause acne. Acne is caused by excessive oils plugging up skin pores.

In conclusion, it is impossible to present in these few pages all of the helpful tips for parenthood. As a parent, no matter how much you have learned and how well you nurture your children, you will make mistakes. Believe it or not, children survive, forgive their parents, and progress to adulthood to become parents themselves.

Any "retribution" for us parents comes when the wonderful cycle of life comes around again in the form of grandchildren!

References

1. Immunization Action Coalition, 1573 Selby Avenue, St. Paul, MN 55104.

2. Rudolph, Abraham M. *Pediatrics*, (Norwalk, CT: Appleton & Lange, 1987).

3. Schmidt, B. O. *Your Child's Health*, (New York: Bantam Books).

WHEN CHILDREN AND TEENS NEED SHOTS

AGE	Hep-B Hepatitis B	DTP* Diphtheria, Tetanus, Pertussis	Hib* Haemophilus influenza type b	OPV Polio	MMR Measles, Mumps, Rubella	Chickenpox Varicella
BIRTH	💉					
2 MONTHS	💉	💉	💉	💉		
4 MONTHS		💉	💉	💉		
6 MONTHS	💉	💉	💉			
2-15 MONTHS		💉	💉		💉	💉
4-6 YEARS		💉		💉	💉 May be given at 4-6 years or 11-12 years	
11-12 YEARS	All teens need 3 hepatitis B shots 💉💉💉	Just diphtheria and tetanus, not pertussis 💉				💉
14-16 YEARS						

* Sometimes the DTP and the Nib are given together in one shot.   ** Depending on the brand, this dose of Hib may not be needed.

The above chart shows the earliest commonly recommended ages for giving vaccines. Your doctor or nurse may have a slightly different schedule, so check with your clinic. If you don't have a clinic, contact your local health department.

Health Maintenance Checklist
for Adults

— Total and HDL cholesterol checked every five years beginning at age twenty.

— Blood pressure checked at least once a year.

— Get regular aerobic exercise.

— Quit smoking if you have the habit.

— Get a tetanus vaccine every ten years, to prevent lock-jaw in case of injuries becoming infected with this particular organism.

— Get the pneumococcal (pneumonia) vaccine once at age sixty-five, or earlier if you have a chronic disease such as lung diseases, diabetes, or sickle cell anemia.

— Have a digital rectal exam for colon cancer screening each year, beginning at age forty.

— Have a fecal occult blood test for colon cancer screening each year beginning at age fifty.

— Have a flexible sigmoidoscopy for colon cancer screening every three to five years beginning at age fifty.

Women only:

— Have a baseline mammogram at age thirty-five, every two years between ages forty to forty-nine, yearly at age fifty and over.

— Do a breast self-exam each month.

165

— Have an annual PAP smear beginning at age eighteen, or when sexual intercourse first begins, whichever comes first.

Men only:

— Have a prostate exam every year beginning at age forty.

— Get a PSA blood test for prostate cancer annually beginning at age fifty.

This list is for healthy adults with no symptoms of disease and for those with normal test results. If any test turns out abnormal, follow-up should be as directed by a physician, not by this chart.

In addition to health, other areas of life which African-Americans need to examine include education, communication, and political-economical. A healthy body needs a healthy mind and a healthy social climate in which to live and operate.

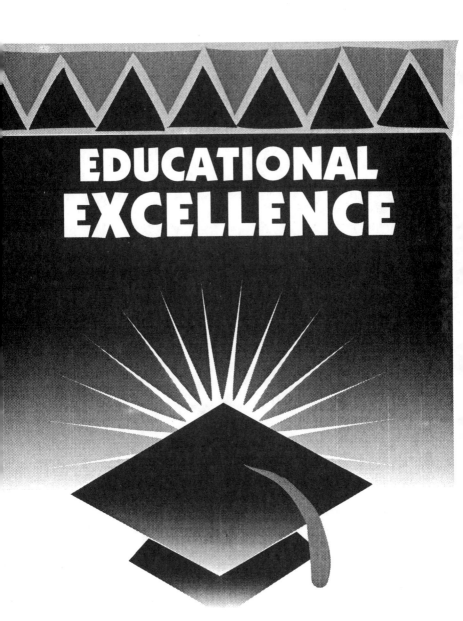

EDUCATIONAL
EXCELLENCE

A Good Education Begins in Childhood

by A. Maria Newsome, M.D.

In this era of incredible technological advances, such as space exploration, heart transplants, and test-tube babies — just to name a few — a strong education is unquestionably the key to an exciting and financially rewarding future.

A good education first begins with wise parents who have the insight to stimulate and challenge their children at an early age. It continues with the fundamental knowledge learned in elementary school and picks up momentum with the more difficult, yet essential, skills learned in high school and beyond.

A generation ago, the average American was able to make a good living by possessing physical strength, dedication, and determination. Today, high-tech machinery has replaced muscle power, and computers have eliminated the need for many jobs altogether.

Consequently, being successful in today's job market requires a person to grow along with society's advancing needs and rapidly increasing information. Today's most advanced technological equipment is tomorrow's antique.

Training beyond the high school level often is the sole difference between those who struggle to pay for food and shelter and those who struggle to pay for beautiful homes and expensive automobiles. Practically everyone has to work hard in life. The main difference is the kind of work each does and the salary received for doing it.

Most jobs that do not require special skills, such as flipping burgers or mopping floors, do not provide good pay or good benefits. Many are "dead-end," boring positions offering neither financial security nor a chance of significant advancement.

These days, competition for the good jobs is stiff. It is extremely difficult to "climb the ladder of success" without a good education.

After all, running a successful business in America's highly competitive market requires much more than great physical skill. It requires knowledge of a variety of aspects of accounting, management, and advertising. Paramount is a working knowledge of computers and data processing systems.

Nevertheless, in many respects, the average manual laborer works harder than the businessman who employs him.

His feet swell from standing, his hands are rough and blistered, his back aches from bending and lifting, and his joints and muscles cry out for their next five-minute break. He gets soaked with April's showers, scalded by August's heat, and is frostbitten by December's spine-tingling chills.

While he is working so hard by the sweat of his brow, his superiors are using their minds instead of physical labor to make a living. They wear designer suits and sit behind comfortable desks, sheltered from the wilds of Mother Nature by the thermostat within arm's reach. They spend their days in deep thought, ever trying to improve the efficiency of their companies or making lucrative deals with wealthy clients.

This does not mean that white collar workers do not work hard in a different way. Their days also are filled with hard work and their nights with stress and uncertainty. Many have to contend with medical problems created by job stress, such as tension headaches, stomach problems, and high blood pressure.

The point is that, because of their better educations, usually they receive much higher salaries and better benefits than their blue collar co-workers. There is no question that educational background often is the only distinguishing factor between two people with similar levels of intelligence leading very dissimilar lifestyles.

Early Blacks Had No Educational Opportunities

As most people know, there was a long period in American history when it was illegal for slaves to get an education and for anyone to teach them. They were only taught enough of the language to obey orders.

They were brought to this country from Africa like animals, shackled together tightly in sweltering cargo holds. Diseases spread so rapidly through those "hell-holes" that many died long before reaching their destination. Others committed suicide in any way they could rather than be stripped of their freedom and dignity.

African men were relegated from being proud leaders and providers to being mere property, beaten into submission like beasts of burden.

African women were robbed of self-respect through beatings and rapes. They were bred and auctioned off like cattle, as if families did not exist. Parents and children, husbands and wives, brothers and sisters were separated and sold and many never saw their loved ones again.

When they arrived in this country, they had no formal education and no knowledge of the English language at all. (See the section on Communications.)

In addition, there was much mixing of the races through white men raping black women. The proof of this becomes painfully apparent when one compares the appearance of the average African-American with the average African today.

Most blacks brought to America as slaves were intelligent and yearned for knowledge, but were forced to educate themselves in secret. Not knowing the language or customs and being thrown into a totally different culture *as slaves and inferiors* caused them to appear unintelligent to whites.

In addition, the trauma of this transition from Africa to the southern United States did irreparable damage to the emotions and personalities (self-esteem and self-confidence) of most slaves.

Those who wanted to learn to read English had to hide in back rooms, while others served as look-outs. There were a few exceptions made for slaves trained to do household accounts. However, no slave with any "get up and go," any personal pride, was allowed any education for fear they would get "uppity."

If most of the slaves tried to get even a rudimentary education and were discovered, they faced beating, or sometimes, even death. This inhumane treatment was to intimidate other slaves who might try to do the same thing.

However, despite the tremendous threat to their lives and well-being, many brave Africans refused to yield to their oppressors' wishes to ignore their God-given intelligence and pressed on with the search for knowledge.

A strong education for black Americans was a priority of our forefathers who fought and died for our human and civil rights. The struggle was long, and the price was high. Blood was shed, but lives were willingly laid down so that future generations of African-Americans could have the right to obtain a high quality education comparable to that available to white Americans.

Our ancestors had the insight to realize how important

a good education is to success. Despite constant "brainwashing" to the contrary, they had enough wisdom and pride to know that the intellectual potential of a black American was as high as that of any other American when given an equal opportunity.

Many doors have been opened for this generation of blacks by the tremendous sacrifices of past generations, who fought for a better future for the African-American race. If we as a race plan to move forward, we must learn to take much better advantage of the opportunities available to us than we do at present.

As more black individuals become highly successful and political pressure increases to phase out affirmative action programs, things will change. There will be no understanding of, or allowance for, any deficiencies whatsoever, whether they are the result of a disadvantaged background or not.

Blacks must be, in every way, as competitive as their white counterparts who seek the same positions — and if the prospective employer has racist tendencies, even more so.

Unfortunately, black youth are dropping out of high schools in record numbers. As a result, many extremely intelligent young blacks are finding themselves on welfare, in low-paying jobs, unemployed, or involved in some illegal activity in order to make money. Meanwhile, other races of people are continuing to complete high school, college, and professional schools in high numbers.

As long as this trend continues, a high percentage of blacks will remain economically and socially disadvantaged, while men and women of other races continue to be the bosses. This gap will not be because those other races are smarter, but because they are better prepared to meet society's demands.

Furthermore, a frighteningly large percentage of African-American children are being born to young, single mothers who have neither experienced economic nor educational success for a variety of reasons. Due to a lack of personal experience in these areas, many good, well-meaning mothers will have great difficulty selling their own children on the importance of a good education.

As a result of starting at a disadvantage and having to compete with the many negative influences children of the 90s face, many mothers will be unsuccessful in their attempts to motivate their children to excel in school.

In an era of "alternative success" through such things as selling drugs, many of these brilliant children will be lured into destructive activities in an attempt to find respect while making money.

People Cannot Be Forced to Learn

These depressing scenarios do not have to continue to come true and even escalate!

Although it is true that the Afro-American race would not be in its present predicament had it not been for slavery and racism, it is essential to recognize that there will *never* be a great politician, black or white, who can undo the numerous psychological, social, and economic effects of centuries of racism. If we intend to progress and prosper, it will only come through our own efforts.

This is not to say that we can do everything without political power. It simply means we have to take the lead in our own lives, not remain passive bystanders who have no choice but to "roll with the punches."

If we plan to turn the tide on the present state of affairs in the black community, we each need to get involved in the struggle on an individual basis.

First of all, that means voting and encouraging everyone we know to register and vote for the politicians and school board members who will set policies that will best benefit our children's education.

For example, there is heated controversy over whether to incorporate black history into everyday history books, and not just leave it up to Black History Month events.

Children of all races need to know the truth about the black race. When I was in grade and high school, I only learned about the late Civil Rights leader, Martin Luther King, Jr., about the scientist-inventor George Washington Carver, and about the many, many slaves. Consequently, my perception of black achievements was extremely limited. It seemed as if all the heroes were white.

However, when I took black history courses in college, I was stunned to find out about the many great accomplishments of blacks which authors of public school history textbooks had chosen to omit.

Black children desperately need to know how they fit into the scheme of the world. White children learn about hero after hero who was white. This serves as a tremendous source of racial pride and satisfaction. On the other hand, black children are not taught about black heroes to any comparable extent.

By picking and choosing which great stories to tell and which ones to omit, educators have had a tremendous impact. On the one hand, they have perpetuated racism and, on the other, fostered low self-esteem among blacks.

White children are not born viewing themselves as superior to blacks, and black children are not born viewing themselves as inferior to whites. These views must be learned.

Unless the structure of public education is changed to accommodate the needs of all races, future generations of children will continue to be fed limited information on the history of the world.

Not only will white children continue to be deceived into believing that blacks have added little to civilization, but black children also will believe this falsehood.

The end result is that both races will lose, because this subconscious programming of the way one views one's own race compared to other races only serves to perpetuate many, many social ills. For example, as I wrote earlier, many children in public schools do not realize that many of the ancient Egyptians, whose great pyramids revolutionized the fields of math and science, had very dark skins.

Public libraries have numerous books on Egypt, which are full of photographs, drawings, and artwork showing ancient Egyptians as beautiful, brown-skinned people, even in some self-portraits that have lasted into the 20th century. After all, Egypt is in Africa.

I have an Egyptian-born friend who told me that he was amazed when he saw how Egyptians were depicted in American movies. The actors and actresses playing Egyptians usually are Caucasians with a little tanning make-up, while real Egyptians today run the gamut from very fair skin to very dark skin, similar to the range of skin color of African-Americans.

And, judging from the ancient art that has been found, the color of the ancient Egyptians was even more a uniform and darker brown. This friend also said that, contrary to the image portrayed of blacks in America, the dark-skinned people in Egypt are "stereotyped" as being the nicest and the most kind.

Despite the tremendous inspiration most people feel while watching Charlton Heston play Moses in that great epic film, *The Ten Commandments*, there is a great discrepancy between Scripture and screenplay — as is true most of the time when Hollywood decides to "rewrite God" and dramatize the Bible!

Among literary figures who have at least some black ancestry, one of the foremost was Alexandre Dumas, grandson of a black woman from the Dominican Republic, who wrote the classics, *The Count of Monte Cristo* and *The Three Musketeers* (now known by most children as the name of a candy bar, not a famous book)! His father was one of Napoleon's generals and his son wrote a famous play, *Camille*.

The list of little known but highly noteworthy achievements by people of black ancestry is very long. However, as long as so many American schools do a very poor job of educating students about the accomplishments of all races, every student will be cheated out of valuable information that could help him become a better, more well-rounded person.

Separate But Equal Was Not "Equal"

Even after the Civil War ended and the Fourteenth Amendment was passed giving slaves freedom, little provision was made for the educating of their children. It was almost thirty years before education for blacks became part of our legal system.

The *Plessy vs. Ferguson* decision of 1896 upheld the "separate but equal" doctrine that stated it was okay to have separate facilities for blacks and whites as long as they were equal.

A half-century later, the settling of another case finally brought the admission from the federal court system that, actually, school facilities for blacks and whites were extremely *unequal*.

Educating black children until the 1950s was not taken as seriously as educating white children. Black children were thought to have low intelligence quotients and to not be capable of learning as much as their white counterparts.

Black schools had poorer buildings, and teachers were

paid less. Black schools could not offer their students the same potential for learning. They were not allocated funds for the same high quality learning materials that were given to white schools.

Furthermore, there were not many well-educated black teachers (hence the rationale for lower salaries).

Most adults had fallen prey in their own generation to the same racist attitudes and forces that hindered blacks from obtaining good educations. Therefore, the poor-education syndrome was perpetuated through several generations, even after Emancipation.

As a result of the landmark decision in the case of *Brown vs. the Board of Education*, Topeka, Kansas, in 1954, the federal government acknowledged that black children were not receiving an adequate education, much less an equal one. The U.S. Supreme Court called for the integration of all public schools in this decision.

However, in spite of the mandate from the nation's highest court, proceedings did not move smoothly. There was intense opposition, often extending to actual violence, from whites who objected to the presence of black students in traditionally white schools.

Even today, two generations later, many white learning institutions use subtle measures to limit the number of blacks attending or from successfully completing their programs of study.

This on-going hostility shows up in the increasing number of incidents of racial violence on college campuses nationwide. Furthermore, many predominantly black schools — whether inner-city grade schools or black colleges — do not receive the same funding as do white schools.

The point is that throughout American history, most blacks have not had the same educational opportunities as whites. This lack of a comparable education, accompanied by the numerous negative psychological and social factors to which blacks are exposed, make an unholy climate that works to hold blacks back.

Children, as well as adults, must be given a reason to learn.

Give Students a Reason to Learn

Everyone has the need to feel accepted and liked by others, but children are particularly vulnerable to peer pressure. Unfortunately, the lack of the kind of familiarity which brings comfort in a certain situation, may cause black parents and friends to ridicule those who try to excel in academics.

Many African-Americans have "bought into" the belief that education and good language habits are for whites, not blacks. We seem to have embraced this prejudice against us and made it our own thinking.

Most blacks do not realize that when they come against a good education or properly spoken English, they are saying, "Yes, Mr. White Man, you were right about us. We'll just be proud of our poor education and poor language skills because, after all, *it is our 'thing' to do this.*"

Although students of all races are susceptible to being called "nerds" in some places if they get top grades and are very "bookish," African-American students sometimes have to deal with an extra portion of this resentment from their peers.

For instance, when a black youth speaks English correctly, his peers often insult him although he is not even using "big words" or difficult phrases. They accuse him of "trying to be white."

However, it is racist to associate the use of good English with whites and the use of bad English with blacks, no matter which race is perpetuating that falsehood.

Unfortunately, this example demonstrates only one manifestation of the deeply rooted negativism and lack of understanding many blacks have toward academic excellence.

When a child is harassed for getting good grades in school and behaving well, he often changes these good habits into bad ones. However, when children are surrounded with other children who are high achievers, they will not be teased for doing well.

So many white Americans are well-educated and successful that they know what it takes to achieve high goals and are able to pass this wisdom on to their children.

Also, many white children plan from an early age to go to college as do many of their friends. This serves as a tremendous reinforcement for children from parents, peers, and other societal entities.

On the other hand, many African-Americans are outwardly intolerant of the racism that hinders the success of black people, while saying and doing things that tear down or hinder their black friends from pursuing academic success.

The average white American student these days faces many potential obstacles to his success, and the average black student faces even more.

There is no way we can encourage the young minds of our children, while expecting them to overcome such a tremendous psychological obstacle as anti-academic or anti-language excellence pressure from their peers and from many adults as well.

Parents are the first line of defense against defeat. There are many things parents can do to guide their children in the right educational direction. Parents must take a strong and unwavering stand about the importance of education. Their roles must be active and not just passive. It is one thing to preach to a child about the importance of his education. It is another to lead by example.

If the parents spend all of their spare time in front of the television set, never engaging in any intellectually stimulating activities themselves, any spoken message they give their children on the importance of learning will undoubtedly be less effective.

For example, those parents who have never finished high school could take GED courses and work toward getting a high school equivalency diploma. That does not take very much time, energy, or money compared to the results it could bring in the job market. Also, it would send a powerful message to their children about the importance of cultivating the mind.

Another way in which parents can have a very positive influence on their children's attitude to education is to encourage them to read in their spare time.

In this era of video games and cable television, children often are tempted to engage in mindless activities. Most children will shy away from things that develop their minds anyway, if not influenced and encouraged to a great extent.

Children Need To Learn Black History

Books can be checked out from the local public library at no expense, so there is no reason a child should not have access to a world of knowledge. Parents can foster this by spending some of their own spare time reading.

Encouraging reading can have two purposes: developing a well-informed and educated mind and learning about black history. Children should be pointed in the direction of books and programs that teach them about our ancestors and our black heritage. At this point in time, many books on black history are available that are geared toward various age groups.

If possible, parents should invest a few dollars in buying some of these books to keep at home so children can read them over and over. When black children go to school, usually they will not learn about all of the important accomplishments of their ancestors.

Instead, they will learn how important whites have been throughout history and that the traditional place of the black person has always been below that of whites.

This generation of African-Americans must make it a top priority to provide our children with the best possible opportunities for learning. This not only requires instilling a desire in them to want to learn, but it requires good school teachers. It requires good home teaching as well.

Even before a child reaches kindergarten years, parents can actively work at developing that child's mind through learning toys.

A variety of games are available that turn learning into fun and give a child a head start on developing a variety of important developmental and intellectual skills which they will soon need. These educational tools stimulate and challenge little minds while providing them with entertainment.

The confidence provided by a good education and the knowledge of the worth of our black ancestors to society will go a long way toward rebuilding self-esteem and a feeling of self-worth into our children.

The African-American child has very special needs that go beyond those of his non-black classmates. He needs extra strength and emotional support to help him prepare to successfully endure the many challenges he will face in school, as well as life in general.

Parents, family members, and even friends of those with small children should make extra efforts to instill a sense of pride in black ancestry in them.

The ongoing controversy about Eurocentric versus Afrocentric curricula in public schools may never end in our children being taught by an Afrocentric curriculum. Nevertheless, parents should begin teaching their children at an early age about the historical contributions of Africans and African-Americans.

Regardless of how this information is obtained, developing pride in the black race should be a priority in the home of every African-American. An early education about the numerous noteworthy contributions blacks have made to the world, even in the face of enormous oppression, can play a very instrumental role in developing a strong sense of racial pride and self-respect.

It is inevitable that, as a black child grows up, he or she will see many African-Americans living in poverty, unemployed, or employed in low-paying, dead-end jobs.

Furthermore, he will probably be confronted by peers who try to convince him that his blackness is an insurmountable obstacle to "traditional" success. Consequently, they may try to tempt him into seeking prosperity and "respect" through dealing drugs or some other criminal activity.

However, if that child already has a deep-rooted self-respect and strong attitude toward improving himself to compete in society for the better jobs, he will be more likely to withstand the powerful persuasion of those temptations.

If he truly believes in the strength and beauty of the black race in general, and in himself in particular, he will be better prepared to overcome the seduction and danger of living a fast but often short life.

Faith in God and Belief in Oneself

By beginning with the love and standards of God Almighty, even children come to realize that there is a power higher than themselves. This can be extremely crucial both early and late in a child's life.

Although a young child may not totally understand

the language or meaning of parts of the Bible, he can still develop an understanding of its basic meaning. Also, there are several modern-language versions available today.

Knowing that God loves all children equally and that no one has power over God gives a person a kind of personal empowerment that no one can take away. No matter what happens to his parents, he can know that God always will be there.

That is a very important starting point for life, a foundation that many of our ancestors stood on in order to endure and to accomplish the things they did.

Our ancestors may not have had access to education, but most of them did have access to God. It was considered not only okay but almost mandatory to expose slaves to the Bible and to God. Our black spirituals reflect the help God became to them, a very present help in all times of need.

Getting a child established in a good church is more important than getting him or her into a good school. It also is important for children to know that their parents believe in them. It is crucial for parents to demonstrate unwavering faith in their children's abilities, both intellectual and creative.

Although many families cannot afford expensive pre-school programs or high-tech learning aids such as computers, most parents do have an intense desire to help their children succeed in life. It is this desire that will do the most to foster within them a love of learning and a desire to succeed.

Children blindly follow their parents' guidance up to a certain age. The psychological implications of the direction they receive — good or bad — cannot be overestimated. Even as adults, we crave support and comfort from those we love, but children have an even greater need.

If a child's parents show that they believe he is smart

and capable, and if they encourage him always to do his best, that child will have a strong built-in drive for accomplishment. The feeling of pride that comes from praise and attention from parents will be transmuted into a pride in self-accomplishment.

Parents should greet A's and B's with special attention and lots of praise. This is not to say that parents should expect straight A's from every child every time. It can do as much damage to chastise a child for not living up to expectations as not to encourage him at all.

A C for some children may be their best, and even A students may not make A's all the time in every subject. Different children learn at different rates and have different intellectual capacities. Parents should encourage a child to do his best, seek out the means by which to help him reach his potential, and then respect his limitations.

Most children, with strong motivation, hard work, and good teaching can do well in school. On the other hand, if a child works hard and gets no appreciation, no matter what grades he makes, he may feel no need to strive for good grades but feel satisfied with only passing grades.

If parents do not provide that initial boost for the child to excel, it will be extremely difficult for any teacher to fill that void, no matter how good his teaching methods. Children must be propelled by something within.

Homework is one area of school life that shows quickly where a child's motivation lies.

Children Need Immediate Rewards

By nature, children love to have fun. Most of them do not understand the importance of studying on a beautiful day when they really want to be outdoors playing with their friends or just lounging around on the sofa watching their favorite television programs. It is only natural for a child to try to rush through homework to get into more "fun" activities.

Children deal in the here and now. They live in the present, with the past remote and the future unknowable, unimaginable. Neither do they understand abstract concepts, such as delayed gratification: Work today so that you can enjoy tomorrow. Most children work harder if there is an immediate reward involved.

Personally, I was the type of child who liked to have fun after school and did not want to study very much. My parents frequently offered monetary incentives for getting good grades, such as 50 cents for every A and a quarter for every B on my report cards.

Ideally, I should have wanted to do well for the personal sense of accomplishment. However, I must confess that monetary stimulus strengthened my motivation to study when I otherwise would have chosen to play.

However, even more motivating than the few dollars I earned for a good performance were the praise and the attention I received from my parents. This encouragement was extremely instrumental in building a high self-esteem in me and molding a positive self-image.

Furthermore, that look of pride and satisfaction on their faces was a much more welcome sight than the dreaded look of disappointment when I did not bring home the grades I should have, causing them to know that I had been slacking off. My own feelings of discontent and regret only added to my guilt.

Regardless of how I did on any particular grading period, I realized at a very young age that I *could* achieve high levels when I put my mind to it. There were many times during my higher education days when I looked back on those early years and received a great sense of reinforcement of my personal abilities.

When classes became tough I remembered how I had always been able to do as well as my classmates of all races when I really applied myself. I learned early that getting bad grades was an option, a choice, just as much as getting good grades. It depended on my personal level of commitment. There were times, however, when I had to remind myself that I was just as smart as anyone else.

One very potent result of underachievement is poor self-esteem. If a child does poorly in school, whether due to lack of stimulation or to special learning needs, and comes to view himself as "stupid," he may just give up on learning.

If a child brings home C's and D's, his parents should not insult him and make him feel stupid. Certainly, they should never call him "stupid." That is a self-fulfilling "prophecy." He will become what he is called, because he believes his parents speak truth.

If he does believe them, what will be his motivation for even trying to do well?

If he sincerely believes he is unintelligent, what will inspire him to hurdle particularly difficult subjects like math and science?

Since even the smartest students have difficulty with these hard courses, how can he expect to compete with them intellectually when he is handicapped by such a tremendous psychological burden?

In this kind of home situation, a child often gives up before he really begins. If he does not believe in himself, he may very well choose to save himself the letdown and humiliation of failure by not trying in the first place.

At least that way, when he fails, he will not feel as much pain and disappointment as he would if he had given it his best shot but failed anyway.

A parent should never, under any circumstances,

simply assume that a child is not intelligent and accept poor grades as "the best that can be expected."

In a large percentage of cases, poor academic performance does not truly reflect a lack of intelligence. There may be some other unidentified reasons for his poor performance such as lack of stimulation from home.

Even if a parent did not excel in academics himself, that is no indication that his children are not intellectually capable of succeeding either. If that parent's own parents had understood how to motivate him and enhance his educational experience, he might have excelled.

Considering the social, economic, and racial climate of America during his upbringing and the probable inability of his own folks to provide him with a high quality education, no wonder his own achievements were low.

Many adults working today as janitors who dropped out of school might have been college graduates if they had been given the proper guidance and the right opportunities.

Nipping Problems in the Bud

Poor grades in the first couple of years of school do not necessarily mean a child will be a high school dropout. However, those grades do need to be addressed and early. If a child is doing poorly in the easy grades, there is a good chance he will fall so far behind that he will find it extremely difficult to catch up.

If he fails to gain the basic skills taught in the early grades, he will fall even further behind. The more advanced grades build more and more on that fundamental knowledge base that should have been built in the first years of school.

The underlying cause of his problem needs to be discovered. Some children do have learning disabilities that require special attention. If this is discovered early, and the child gets the help he needs to overcome the disability, his chances for a favorable outcome are much higher than if this disability were never discovered or even was found at a later stage.

Perhaps the child needs glasses or a hearing aid, or perhaps his health is such that he is not able to concentrate well. Poor nutrition makes a poor student.

Parents should talk to their child and to his teacher to determine what the problems are and how they may be solved. They should find out the child's strengths and weaknesses and make a serious attempt to cultivate the strengths and strengthen the weaknesses.

It would be good to ask both teacher and child for specific advice on how to help the child understand the material better and how he could study more efficiently.

It may simply require a stricter study schedule, such as setting aside two or three uninterrupted hours of studying each evening, and sticking to it. Alternatively, the child may benefit from a variety of study aids that can be cheaply purchased from any bookstore.

On the other hand, perhaps he could benefit from personal tutoring by a family member, a friend, or even a hired tutor. There are numerous ways a concerned parent can improve his child's educational outcome. However, he must diligently seek answers and not give up if the first method tried proves not to work.

Regardless of how a child is doing in school, the parent-teacher relationship is a crucial one. The teacher should be comfortable enough to tell parents when their child needs help and how they can go about giving him the assistance he needs. Likewise, the teacher should be able to tell parents when a child is or is not working up to his potential and when he needs to be disciplined.

When a child knows his parents and teachers are working together productively, he will not try to play them against each other. The same is true of parents. They should not let the children play them against one another.

A child needs to know that he cannot use the excuse, "I got a bad grade because the teacher doesn't like me."

Furthermore, he will be more likely to behave if he knows he will be sent to the principal's office if he acts up and that his teacher will contact mom and dad as well. Perhaps he would have another punishment waiting when he gets home — a double incentive for good behavior.

Unfortunately, the parent-teacher relationship does not always run so smoothly. As a matter of fact, there is often tremendous animosity between them.

When children do not appear to be learning, many parents automatically point a finger of blame at the teachers, as if it were all their fault. Teachers are not magicians, although it is important for them to be able to motivate children and make learning fun.

When parents fail to provide their children with the primary motivation to learn or fail to teach them to respect their teachers, they cannot realistically expect the teacher to turn out a rocket scientist.

Learning Never Occurs Without Discipline

In today's society, discipline problems are commonplace. One good thing about the old schools was that students respected teachers. We may have better educational standards today, but because of lax discipline in many homes and permissiveness by school policy in many places, respect for teachers has eroded.

Some twenty years ago, the focus in education moved away from learning and onto allowing the students to learn "self-expression." True self-expression requires self-discipline.

It used to be a very daring thing for students to run down the hall or chew gum in class. Today, teachers as well as students fear physical violence. Some children even carry guns at school and are not afraid to use them if the mood strikes.

A recent article about stress-related careers in America listed inner-city school teaching as more stressful than being a doctor or even a policeman. Children have absolutely no business intimidating any adult, especially a teacher who is trying to help them succeed in life. A teacher cannot function efficiently when students do not respect him or her or pay attention.

However, *discipline should be the responsibility of parents, not teachers.*

Teachers spend years and energy in college to learn how to provide their students with a quality education to help prepare them to succeed in life. There are plenty of higher paying, more glamorous fields which they could have chosen. Teaching is a "service" profession. Most teachers genuinely want to contribute to the success of America's youth and America's future.

Teachers deserve tremendous respect and appreciation for their efforts. They were not trained as "police," nor do they deserve the responsibility of disciplining disrespectful and sometimes dangerous youth.

Yesterday's disciplinary problems were solved by sending students to the principal's office. Today, students talk back to their teachers, and some even scare teachers into doing nothing by threats of violence. Furthermore, the parents of a child sent to the principal's office for discipline may become angry at the principal!

Although there always will be a small percentage of parents who put their responsibility on the teacher and expect a teacher to fulfill the unrealistic role of both parent and educator, many parents do personally struggle against the influences of society. Checking up on their own children will not solve the juvenile problems in American society, but it is a positive and productive step forward. If more parents took this responsibility seriously once again, schools would run much more smoothly and efficiently.

Another reason for building a good working relationship with one's children's teachers is the fact that a small percentage of teachers pass their students on to the next grade when they really have not adequately learned the skills they need to succeed in more advanced classes. Others do not set high enough requirements for the grades they assign.

For example, a young twelve-year-old friend of mine wrote an English paper entitled, "Why Black Males Are an Endangered Species."

Although he made numerous basic grammatical, spelling, and punctuation errors, he received an "A" on his paper. His teacher did not bother even marking all of the errors.

Consequently, in his mind, there was no need for improvement. He really believed he was doing "A," or excellent, work. Had he submitted the same paper to a teacher in a suburban junior high school, he unquestionably would have received a "C" or lower on account of so many basic English errors on an English assignment, no matter how good the content and concepts of the essay were.

It is not fair to children in the long run to allow them to get away with not learning the things for which they are supposedly getting good grades. If they do not realize their deficiencies early and work to improve them, they will fall further and further behind.

An inferior education is a large price to pay for avoiding embarrassment for not keeping up with one's peers.

All parents need to be sure their children really are learning and not just "passing." Many who "just pass" will pay for their teachers' and parents' leniency by being forced to take low-paying, dead-end jobs.

Despite their initial drive and spirit, some will fall prey eventually to the seduction of the "easy money" they could make in illegal activities.

The pain of being stuck in a job that is neither intellectually stimulating nor financially rewarding but just drudgery while seeing others with exciting, great paying careers can be overwhelming. Always, there will be those who, in hopes of temporarily escaping their humdrum existence, give in to the deceptive enticement of drugs and alcohol.

These chemical substances will become their way of coping with dreary, unhappy lives. Unfortunately, many realize when it is too late that they have traded in harmless boredom for a seemingly inescapable nightmare of chemical addiction. This ever-increasing roller coaster of psychological and physical dependence coupled with its accompanying financial ruin and broken families, further intensifies the cycle of depression and unhappiness.

Others end up on welfare with several children. Although they may have been young when they had the babies, growing up and looking for a better life for themselves and their children exposes them to the fact that they are not qualified for challenging jobs. Often, these women find the jobs for which they are qualified would not even pay for a babysitter to look after the children while they work.

Others simply hear complaints about the lack of good

paying jobs and never even attempt to do better. They give up without trying.

The Need To Make Expectations Realistic

Most young people have absolutely no realistic insight into future financial responsibilities. They are unable to fully understand how difficult it is to make a living because for many, their sole income comes in the form of allowances and hand-outs from their parents.

Even if they have a part-time job after school, usually they use that money for extras like clothes and recreation. The burden of providing food and shelter still lies on the parents' shoulders.

Many young people are deceived by music videos and television shows that depict young people driving expensive cars, living in beautiful homes, and having lots of money. Too many of them believe they too can easily acquire these things.

What they fail to realize is that the type of job that pays the salaries required to live that way are extremely hard to get without a good education.

Recently, some friends and I spoke to a remedial class of black high school students about the importance of getting a good education. We were speaking to a group of students who had failed the basic English requirements needed to move on to the next grade. Several of them were years behind their peers.

Unfortunately, in spite of being held back, several of them were even failing this remedial class. They just did not care about learning.

However, when we questioned them about the lifestyles they planned to have, all of them wanted nice, expensive things. Some even wanted six-figure homes and luxurious cars. Yet they were not applying themselves enough to even graduate from high school, much less be prepared to enter the type of post-graduate educational programs they would need to be able to afford these things sometime in the future.

They had great difficulty separating fact from fantasy. The blind spot was not seeing a connection between education and realizing their dreams. One young man wanted to play professional football, yet his grades would not even get his foot in the door of a university these days. Nevertheless, in his mind, his athletic abilities were all he needed to become rich and famous.

A couple of other young men hinted subtly at the fact that they would make their fortunes by dealing drugs. Several young ladies had no idea how to become rich, but they were determined they would do so.

Countless numbers of American youth, especially minority children, are becoming more and more disenchanted with learning. There are numerous reasons why black students are dropping out of high school, but whatever the reason, those dropouts find out sooner or later that it is not nearly as easy to make an honest, comfortable living without a good education as they once thought.

In spite of eventually realizing this fact, many never choose to return to school for a variety of reasons. They remain among the ranks of the unemployable or underemployed. Their brilliant minds find themselves attached to hands glued to a mop.

It Helps To See Reality in Black and White

In the face of all these misconceptions, parents should make a very serious effort to inform their children realistically about the future they will one day face with or without an education.

One way to give a child a taste of what lies ahead is to roll forward the wheels of time, so to speak, and pretend for a day or so that he is a young adult preparing to venture out into the real world as a responsible, self-sufficient adult.

Practically all young people have a rough idea of the lifestyles they would like to lead. For instance, let us say that a young man tells his parents he plans to live in a beautiful, spacious apartment in a relatively safe neighborhood.

Furthermore, he wants to drive a bright red, convertible sports car, wear the latest fashions, and eat expensive foods. Also, he wants money left over to attend concerts, movies, and other events whenever he pleases.

To make things a little more graphic, a little easier for him to see, his parents might get an apartment guide with colored pictures and apartment layouts. From this, he would get a better idea of how much he would have to pay for apartments of varying sizes and amenities.

These guides usually can be obtained free of charge by calling an apartment locator service, which you may find in a telephone directory just before listings of actual apartments. In this, he could look at apartments ranging from the modest to the luxurious.

Furnishing the apartment he chooses is a task in itself. Visits to several furniture stores to price items or simply looking through catalogs would give him ideas of prices for various qualities of goods.

A careful list of the furniture he chooses, along with the prices, should be kept. Be careful not to overlook the cheaper and less attractive furniture in this overview.

Next, "buy" his dream car. New car brochures can be obtained from dealers, and window shopping is always fun, whether it is serious shopping or just browsing. Actually seeing the cars *and* their prices at dealers' showrooms probably will have a greater impact than just looking at pictures in newspaper ads or magazines.

Perhaps his dream car could be taken for a test drive

with him driving, if he is old enough; if not, as a passenger. Old, run-down, used vehicles also should be covered in this survey so the youth may see the broad range of automobiles from which he may one day be choosing.

His attire is next on the agenda. Young people these days are fashion fanatics. They want to spend more on a pair of tennis shoes than they really ought to be spending on an entire outfit!

Parents should take this child to a mall and let him make a list of what he would buy if he had an unlimited supply of money. This is what many young people think will be the case once they get a job anyway.

In addition to spending an extravagant amount of his imaginary money on clothing, undoubtedly, he would choose a variety of other items including video games, computers, and so forth.

At this point, he has a gorgeous home beautifully furnished, a "flashy" car, and "fresh" clothes. However, even a person as dashing as he needs nourishment. Rummaging through the refrigerator and kitchen cabinets will give him an idea of the cost of food.

Last on the list is recreation. After a hard week on the job, he probably will want to have plenty of fun on weekends. His idea of fun may include taking in a couple of movies, going to cultural exhibits, attending concerts, or even taking out-of-town trips.

The next step is for the parents to sit down with pencil and paper, the Sunday newspaper, and their monthly bills and start figuring out what all of these things will cost. Naturally, prices will vary depending on geographic locations, as well as many other factors.

However, the following *very conservative* sample budget demonstrates the basic principle:

Nice apartment	$400/month
Furniture	100/month
Utilities	50/month
Phone	25/month
Car payment	350/month
Gasoline	40/month
Food, toiletries	175/month
Clothing	100/month
Recreation	50/month
Car Insurance	150/month

Total	$1,440.00 monthly

Our hypothetical youth now knows what things he wants and their approximate cost. If his tastes are expensive, his monthly budget could easily run much higher. Now he needs to figure out how to pay for this desired lifestyle.

Jobs and careers can be projected in the same way as the living expenses. The help-wanted section of Sunday newspapers carries the most comprehensive listings of jobs. Teens should be encouraged to look through the paper and take detailed notes about the jobs they think would meet both personal and financial needs.

This way, it becomes strikingly obvious what types of work are available in today's job market, how much they pay, and what level of experience and education potential employers expect.

Then, to the best of a parent's ability, the youth should be given a brief job description of the positions he has chosen. Emphasis should be placed on job satisfaction and security as much as on the pay scale involved. This will help him understand how he will be spending a large portion of the rest of his life!

After all, as most of us spend a substantial proportion of our lives on our jobs, work plays an enormous role in our overall happiness or lack thereof. If a job provides a person with a sense of personal accomplishment and makes him feel he is respected and needed, he or she will have a high self-esteem and be motivated to do well by many factors.

On the other hand, if a person does not enjoy what he does for a living and does not feel that his work is appreciated or important, a significant part of his life will be taken up by cumbersome tasks with no motivation except mere survival.

Keeping in mind career goals, parents should make sure teens who are "walked through" this lifestyle projection and its cost have realistic expectations for these hypothetical jobs they circle in the newspaper. That means whether or not they plan to finish high school, go on to college and advanced education degrees, or just get any job available.

If a young person plans to finish high school then go to work, help them choose jobs out of the want ads that are open to people with only high school diplomas. Many of the jobs available at this level will be only minimum wage. If someone working at this level only works at one job at a time, he or she should bring home approximately $550 a month.

If he or she wants to quit school and go to work immediately, pick out those jobs available for non-skilled and low-educated employees, such as janitors or fast food restaurant workers. A dropout has an extremely different set of job opportunities than those with either a high school or college education. However, they usually pay only minimum wages as well.

Now, go back to the budget and show all the adjustments that will have to be made considering the potential salary. For example, he may need to find a few roommates to share expenses in order to live in that luxurious apartment.

On a minimum-wage salary, he or she can forget about buying a new sports car. In fact, riding the city bus or catching rides with friends may be the only realistic options. All other expectations also will have to be lowered.

After all the data have been gathered and tabulated, a parent can make an extremely convincing case for not only remaining in school, but for working very hard to get good grades in order to one day be able to choose one's destiny. As long as a young person maintains good grades, he has the power to choose whatever career he wants.

Whether someone wants to be a lawyer, a janitor, or anything in between, he will be able to make that decision if he is a good student. Despite popular belief, even children from low-income households can get a college education. There are numerous financial resources available through both public and private sources to help students finance their education.

However, long before money comes into play, the student must be accepted at an institution of higher learning. Therefore, the primary focus has to be on making good enough grades to be accepted in college in the first place. Practically all colleges, and many technical schools as well, require applicants to take one of the national standardized admissions tests.

Some institutions require the American College Testing Program Test (ACT), while others require the Standard Achievement Test (SAT). These tests are an essential part of the admissions process for a variety of reasons to be discussed in the next article.

A Look at College Entrance Exams

Different schools have a wide diversity of educational and financial resources available to them.

Furthermore, teachers throughout the nation utilize a variety of teaching methods, some of which are much more effective than others. They also have their own standards by which grades are determined.

Students add another dimension to differing educational backgrounds by picking some of their own classes. Therefore, a student who made straight A's easily at one school may have had a very difficult time making B's and C's at another. Likewise, had this student chosen more advanced courses at the same school where he made A's, he might only have made B's and C's.

This great variation in school curricula and the assigning of grades makes it practically impossible for a college admissions committee to accurately compare all American students on the basis of grades alone. Standardized tests eliminate this bias.

As students all over the nation take the same tests, a student's performance relative to the national average and to the performance of other students applying at that particular school, can be judged more fairly.

Students cannot be expected to remember everything learned in previous years. Also, not every little tidbit of information taught in high school is even relevant to determining whether a student possesses the fundamental skills to succeed in more advanced studies.

Therefore, a key purpose of college entrance examinations is to test for knowledge of the crucial skills and the ability to apply them to solve problems and answer questions. These examinations are not easy and should not be taken lightly.

First of all, each person will be competing against very ambitious students throughout the country who will, for the most part, have done a lot of serious preparation. Secondly, college administrators use the test scores as an important criterion in determining whether or not to admit a student.

Thirdly, these scores also are strongly considered in determining who is eligible for certain scholarships and grants as well.

By scoring high, a student not only could get accepted to the college of his choice, he also could increase the opportunities available to him for funding his education. Even if a student has gotten consistently high grades in high school, he should not assume he can breeze through these tests easily. He should take them as seriously as a student who routinely makes C's.

In only a few hours, these examinations are designed to assess knowledge gained during several years of high school training. They are similar to a comprehensive final examination covering years of material, except that only certain concepts and principles are stressed, while others are completely ignored.

Fortunately, there are quite a few highly structured programs and study aids available for students preparing to take these examinations. Most bookstores carry several inexpensive study guides for both the ACT and the SAT (many less than $15). These are invaluable in helping a student prepare.

Many of the educators who write these guides have firsthand knowledge about which principles are stressed on the examinations.

These guides use different approaches. For example, some are organized like textbooks and simply review important concepts. However, some of the more popular study books are made up of several full-length practice tests similar to the actual examination in both type and difficulty of principles stressed, the number of questions asked, and the time allotted to complete them.

At the end of each of these sample tests is a section with detailed explanations of the answers step by step. These explanations give the easiest and quickest way to get the right answer.

They also explain principles and formulas necessary to answer a wide variety of math questions. Therefore, even if a student never even took certain types of math, by remembering a few key concepts and formulas, he could learn how to answer many questions he otherwise would have missed.

One advantage of this method is that students get a lot of practice at working through the same types of questions that will appear on the actual test. Although the actual questions will be different, principles stressed in the preparation books will be basically the same as those stressed on the official exam.

Furthermore, at the beginning of each section is listed the number of questions in that section, as well as the amount of time allotted to finish them. This is also comparable to the amount of time students will be given on the actual test to complete a given amount of work.

Anxiety Can Hinder as Much as Lack of Knowledge

One of the most disabling forces students face when taking a test of this magnitude and importance is *anxiety*. Even a student who has been preparing for six months cannot help but be anxious on the morning of the actual exam.

On the other hand, a student who has not studied enough to know what to expect can reach beyond anxiety into sheer panic. It often appears that the questions must be answered in an incredibly short amount of time.

With no realistic expectations of the number of questions he must answer, or of their complexity, a student could very well "freak out" when he receives the examination. Once someone enters a state of panic, he will not be able to concentrate on anything and often will miss questions that should have been easily answered. By taking and *intensely* studying several practice tests, a student will greatly increase his or her chances of doing well on the official examination.

First of all, he will learn general and specific study tips and test-taking strategies from experts in the field of test preparation. More importantly, he will gain great insight into what he needs to know to score high on the exam.

He will be exposed to important principles over and over again, and this will strengthen these concepts in his mind. Furthermore, he will not only memorize these fundamental principles, he also will learn how to utilize them to answer a wide variety of questions.

Therefore, regardless of how questions are phrased on the actual examination, he will be able to apply the same methodical approaches to get to the right answer, and he will be able to do so efficiently.

Next, he will get a feel for how to budget his time. Many, many students do not finish these examinations before their time is up. Those unfinished questions automatically count the same as if he had answered them and missed them.

If a student practices taking tests over and over, he will develop a strong sense of which questions he can answer correctly in a reasonable amount of time. Then he will know which ones should be put aside to return to after finishing the easier ones.

As the correct answer to a simple question is worth just as many points as the correct answer to a difficult one, why waste a lot of time on any one question? If he gets twenty-two out of thirty correct in one section, the college admissions committee will not know if the eight he missed were easy or difficult. All they will know is his score.

Likewise, a student could concentrate on answering the hard questions and not leave enough time to go back and answer the easy ones. In that case, he might end up with a score much lower than students who knew less than he did.

A student can only optimize his test-taking strategies by practicing taking tests. By seeing the variety of ways in which a concept may be applied, he reinforces his understanding of that concept and his ability to utilize it.

Different individuals learn best in different ways, so each student should experiment to find which way works best for him or her. Many students can buy a study book or two a few months in advance and do very well on the test. Others need a more structured method, which includes professional instruction.

Furthermore, since college admissions scores are used by many scholarship selection committees as one of the criteria for determining which students get cash awards and how much, it would benefit many students to invest more money, as well as more time, on the front end to ensure the best possible results on the tail end.

Educational Centers for Entrance Exams

There are a number of professional test-preparation services available. However the *Stanley H. Kaplan Educational Center Ltd.* is the largest, most experienced test preparation service in the country. The programs offered by this institution are accredited by the Accrediting Commission of the Accrediting Council for Continuing Education and Training, a national accrediting agency listed by the United States Secretary of Education.

These programs are more intense than the ones found in workbooks and study guides. First of all, the programs last several weeks. During that period, students attend several classes with Kaplan's professional instructors.

They not only learn important material but interact freely with the teachers, learning strategies for intelligent guessing when one is not sure of the correct answer. They also learn how to pace themselves to alleviate anxiety and make the most of the time allotted.

In addition, students get home study materials to review in their spare time. I can vouch personally for the value of preparation and for the damage lack of preparation for those entrance exams can do to your hopes for a particular career.

There also are TEST-N-TAPE labs, which I found invaluable when I took their course to prepare for the Medical College Admissions Test (MCAT). These courses include many hours of taped instructions fully explaining countless questions. However, I found that, after having even very difficult concepts explained over and over, they became second nature to me. The first time I took the MCAT, I was not well prepared.

As a result, my score in every area was below the national average. Realizing I did not stand a chance of getting accepted into medical school with those scores, I did not bother to apply.

Luckily, I had heard about the Kaplan course from relatives. My two older brothers had taken it and scored well enough to get into medical school at their first attempts. Also, my sister had taken their law school admissions test course and was accepted into law school on her first try.

Knowing how successful the course had been for them, I decided to take the MCAT preparation course before attempting to take the test again. I spent a great deal of time over the next couple of months listening to the course tapes and making my own notes from them.

Realizing that chemistry was my worst subject, I concentrated most heavily on it. In spite of the fact that I had a job and did not have time to finish all the preparation tapes, the second time I took the MCAT I received a good score in all areas.

Needless to say, after this I did apply to a variety of medical schools and was accepted at most of them. In fact, I ended up turning down interviews.

Ironically, the school where I ended up actually recruited me. They had requested the MCAT scores of minorities in their area of the country, and impressed by my scores, they encouraged me to apply to their institution.

A couple of days after my interview with this school, I received a telephone call telling me I had been admitted. Being very interested in their training program, as well as the financial assistance they were offering, I gladly accepted.

By the grace of God and with the help of the excellent Kaplan training program, I finally was able to realize my dream of training to become a physician. I went from being such a poor candidate for admission to medical school that I did not even waste my time trying to get in to being able to pick between a number of schools.

The Kaplan Educational Centers have a long and successful history of preparing students in all stages of their academic careers to take a variety of important examinations. For example, more than half the students in medical schools today took the Kaplan Medical College Admissions Test course.

Likewise, Kaplan has produced more top scores on the SAT than all other courses combined. Personally, I would highly recommend their program to prepare for any examination.

Naturally these courses are significantly more expensive than the books previously discussed. The ACT course runs $395 and the SAT is $495. However, they do offer scholarships ranging from 10 to 50 percent of the fee, based on financial need. There are approximately 141 Kaplan centers nationwide. For convenience, they are open days, evenings, and weekends to accommodate even the most difficult schedules.

(For additional information, call toll free 1-800-KAP-TEST or look in the local phone book under educational services.)

Unfortunately, despite the many avenues by which a student may seek preparation, many have to take these entrance exams several times because of poor performance. This is not because of low intelligence, but because of inadequate preparation.

Preparation for Exams Is Not "a Rush Job"

Recently, I volunteered to be a math tutor for a short ACT preparation course for some local high school students, most of whom were African-Americans. I have a bachelor's degree in a science field, and engineering calculus was one of my best subjects. Also, I had spent the previous four years studying advanced science in graduate and medical schools.

It never entered my mind that I would have difficulty with high school math. Consequently, I thought I could breeze through teaching this course in no time at all!

Therefore, I waited until the night before the first workshop to work through the practice test I had volunteered to teach. Needless to say, I was not only unable to dash through it, I could barely "waddle" through it! Even worse, I could not finish it in the allotted time.

As a matter of fact, it took me several hours to work through a set of problems that had a time limit of sixty minutes. Even then, there were several questions I simply had to give up on answering. On top of that, I missed a humbling number of answers and ended up spending the entire evening trying to review the material.

I had to get up extra early the next morning to finish reviewing in order to understand the material well enough to be able to explain it to the students. It was not that the test was so difficult. The problem was the fact that it had been so long since I had reviewed *those* principles.

As a result, when I tried to work the sample test, I was neither able to finish it in the allotted time nor to get a respectable number of questions right. However, once I took the time to sit down and read the explanation section thoroughly, most of those principles came back to my memory. The problems became much easier to work, although I have to confess that I still question if I ever had learned some of them.

When I gave the test to approximately 50 high school students the next morning, they all missed the majority of the questions. However, when I went to the chalkboard and worked through the steps it takes to get the right answers, most of them were surprised at how simple many of the concepts were.

A number of those students had never even taken courses such as geometry or trigonometry. They were at a particular disadvantage with certain questions. Even so, once they learned a few basic formulas and principles, they were able to figure out some of the problems.

For four consecutive Saturday mornings, we went through the same scenario. At the beginning of each period, they were given a specific amount of time to work a different sample test. Then they graded their own tests, and we worked through the answers.

Unfortunately, it was rare for a student to get more than half the answers right, even on the last day. Nevertheless, when the principles were explained to them, they felt much more comfortable with working out the problems.

Many of these students had unrealistic expectations of the review course. They actually thought four Saturday mornings of reviewing would be adequate to prepare them to take the most challenging, most important test of their lives.

On the first morning, I asked for a show of hands of those who had an ACT review book. Only two or three raised their hands. Most of those students simply did not realize how invaluable these books are until they saw firsthand how easy it is to fail a test, not from lack of intelligence, but from lack of *recent* exposure to the principles tested.

After that first review session, more of the students purchased a review book to study. However, it was too close to the actual test date for them to be able to fully utilize their books to their greatest ability. I ran into one young man at a store a few months later, and he told me that studying the review book had significantly increased his score over his previous one.

He said that he was going to get an even better review book and start studying it much earlier the next time. He planned to take the test a third time. That young man most likely would not have had to take the test three times, if he had only known how to adequately prepare for the first time.

Unfortunately, African-American students as a race are significantly less prepared to take college entrance exams than they should be. As a result, their test scores do not adequately demonstrate their true intellectual potential.

Nevertheless, with college preparatory books widely available at virtually every bookstore at a cost practically everyone can afford, these low test scores suggest one of two things to college admissions committees:

1. African-American students as a whole do not put forth the time or effort to prepare for these very important tests.

2. They do obtain study materials but cannot master them.

If the first theory is accepted, it implies laziness on the part of black students. If the second prevails, it implies lack of intelligence. Either reason reflects on us as a race.

The following table shows how African-American students have lagged significantly behind other races in college entrance exams:

Scores/Race	1990-91	1991-92	1992-93
SAT-Verbal			
White	441	442	444
Asian-American	411	413	415
American Indian	393	395	400
Mexican-American	377	372	374
African-American	351	352	353
SAT-Mathematical			
Asian-American	530	532	535
White	489	491	494
American Indian	437	432	447
Mexican-American	427	425	428
African-American	385	385	388

Source: College *Entrance Examination Board, National Report on College-Bound Seniors* (various years).

Fortunately, black students' low test scores on college entrance examinations do not reflect intellectual inferiority to other races. They reflect inadequate preparation for the exams. When properly prepared, African-American students can achieve goals as high as any other race of people. Unfortunately, today's students are not adequately enlightened on how to prepare for these tests, nor do they fully understand how the test score can make or break an entire future.

Therefore, it is crucial that blacks in general understand the importance of these tests as well as the avenues by which a student can go about preparing for them. Furthermore, this knowledge needs to be circulated to friends and relatives.

Even strangers — if the situation presents itself —

should be made aware of this situation in order for them to inform their children how to go about scoring high enough not only to get accepted into college but to get scholarships to help finance their education as well.

The key to doing well on these tests is familiarity with specific principles. Since the examinations contain material taught during several years of high school training, the student must realize that he cannot adequately review this enormous amount of material in a week or two. He should begin reviewing several months before the test to give himself ample time to become familiar once more with the material.

It is good to begin early and review gradually so that there is plenty of time at the end of the review period to go back to unclear concepts and study them once again before the actual test. If a student tries to cram such a tremendous amount of material into a couple of weeks before the test, he will only be able to cover a fraction of what he needs to know.

More than likely, he also will get behind in his current school work by trying to spend all of his time at the last minute preparing for an exam for which he will be basically unprepared. He may become extremely stressed out and spend every waking moment reviewing. Even then, the odds would still be greatly against him for waiting so long to begin. Alternatively, when such a student realizes how impossible the task of reviewing this magnitude of information in such a short period of time really is, he may give up on studying for the test altogether and just take his chances.

As a result of the civil rights struggle, there was pressure on universities throughout the country to provide a quality education to minorities. Officials realized that a long history of racism had prevented many generations of blacks from obtaining an education comparable to that given to whites. Therefore, the entrance requirements were set lower for black students than for white students at many institutions, including grades and scores on college entrance examinations.

However, affirmative action programs are now being phased out. Black students of the future will no longer be able to secure college slots if their credentials are not competitive with the ever-increasing standards set by this highly industrialized society.

Tomorrow's black students will have to demonstrate their intellectual potential and determination by grades and standardized test scores alone. Soon there will be no quotas and no legal basis for lawsuits and political pressure against schools that refuse to admit black students or students of any race whose academic performance falls below the standards that each institution has a legal right to set. Consequently, it is crucial that both parents and students understand how to go about preparing for the future.

Guidelines for Parents

by A. Maria Newsome, M.D.

This section is a very concise summary of points for parents who want their children to go to college:

1. Begin by providing good books and a learning atmosphere at home before the child even begins school. This does not have to be expensive and can involve borrowing books from a public library and buying some educational toys for presents instead of all presents being mindless entertainment.

2. Academic excellence should be encouraged at an early age. When a child grows up knowing that when he puts his mind to it, he can accomplish as much as any other child — black, white, Asian, Hispanic, or any other race — he will be much more likely to hang in there during the hard times.

3. Get to know the child's teachers as he or she progresses in school so that you will be on top of any problems before they get out of hand.

When school gets tough, and a child may come to believe he is not smart enough to make it no matter how hard he tries, he will be more likely to take the easy way out, such as switching to easier classes or dropping out altogether.

A teacher usually can spot the beginning of this "dropout syndrome" and alert the parents, if a line of communication has been established. In other words, if the teacher knows the parents are truly interested, he or she will be more likely to become more involved.

215

4. Encourage your child to talk proper English from the very first words he or she learns to say, which means you must use correct English yourself.

5. Get involved in the child's high school curriculum early, preferably at the beginning of the freshman year.

Make sure the guidance counselor knows that your child wants to attend college. Students on a college-bound track are encouraged by counselors to take different classes than those who do not intend to get post-secondary training.

6. If the funds are not there for a child to go to college, parents should begin to look a couple of years ahead for sources that help fund educations for young people. (More details are given later in this article.) Chances are that a child can still go to college, even if his family cannot afford to send him.

7. Months before time to take college entrance exams, a parent can insist that a child get preparatory courses or workbooks and spend time getting ready for the entrance examinations. If possible, a parent should work with the child on reviewing.

Guidance Counselors Can Be Supportive

If the guidance counselor knows not only that a student intends to go to college but also what career he plans to pursue, the counselor will be able to recommend the right courses to help prepare him for his future career. Some of these same classes can also help with preparation for college entrance examinations. For example, if a student wants to become an engineer, his counselor may advise him to take algebra, geometry, trigonometry, and calculus, while most other students are taking fewer, more basic, math courses.

Without this strong background in high school, a student could waste a lot of time and money taking remedial classes when he gets to college. On the other hand, if a student is planning to become a business executive, he would benefit more from math courses geared toward the business field, not toward high-tech science. Consequently, this student's ideal curriculum would be much different from that of the first student's.

Unfortunately, often there is a lack of communication between parents and counselors and between students and counselors as well. The result is that too many students graduate from high school totally unprepared to make their next career move.

As high school students now have a significant input into which courses they want to take, parents ought to know how these choices are going to affect their children in the long run.

Left to their own devices, many students will choose the easiest classes. Most young people are focused on the here and now, not on the rewards they will receive in the future from working hard today.

How many high school students are mature enough to sign up for a difficult class that requires long hours of studying when they can sign up for an easy class that requires little homework?

This mindset of teenagers is totally natural for the growth patterns of those years. At that stage of life, the present is all that is *real* to them. Not all students realize that hard work in high school will pay off in adult life.

Therefore, parents who are serious about their children's academic success will keep an eye on the choices they make for high school classes.

Parents who know the state of mind of teenagers also will take the time to develop relationships with those who teach and guide them in school. Whether those relationships consist of close, personal friendships or simply very productive phone conversations a few times a year, the contact should be made.

If parents do not understand what courses their children should take to best prepare them to reach future goals, how can they effectively encourage children in what courses to take?

Furthermore, if they do not communicate with the teachers, they will not know if a child is working at his true potential. If he is not, without conversations with the teacher, how would they know what the child needs to change or to do differently to improve his performance and enhance his future success?

A child might benefit tremendously from stricter study hours at home, extra study aids or books, or any number of other things. However, if parents do not take time to find out, they will be failing to provide their child with the best possible guidance they can give.

If a student maintains high grades, his chances of not only being accepted into the college of his choice will improve, but as I mentioned earlier, he will have a better chance of qualifying for a variety of educational funding resources to help him pay for his education as well.

His chances in both areas will be much better with good grades than if he just "gets by" in high school.

It is very important for both parents and children to realize that, even if the parents cannot afford college on their own, chances are a child can still go, if they use the right strategies and implement them early enough.

The College Blue Book

Lack of money does not have to be a reason not to pursue higher education. Although the federal government has cut back on some educational grants, it still offers a great deal of financial assistance to those who need it, such as in the form of Stafford loans (previously called Guaranteed

Student Loans).

Furthermore, there are many other extremely important sources available for funding an education. Unfortunately, most people do not realize the tremendous resources available. Therefore, they are not able to utilize them. There are several manuals available which list some of these resources.

For instance, there is a book called *The College Blue Book*, which lists scholarships, fellowships, grants, and loans from literally hundreds of private, institutional, and public sources for educational funding. Look for a current edition of this book at the local library.

This is only one of many books available to those looking for financial assistance with educational expenses. Furthermore, an individual can find all this information absolutely free at the public library.

Just ask the librarian where to find the books on educational financing. Also, many bookstores carry some of these books. Another source is your child's high school counselor. Most counselors keep books with information on educational funding.

However the information is obtained, whether through the library system, the public school system, or a bookstore, this information is invaluable. It can make the difference between a young person's learning how to fry hamburgers and learning how to program rocket ships or computers.

It is extremely important to start very early on these applications.

Institutions, both those who do the funding and those who receive funding, need time to respond to requests for applications and information. It might take weeks just to receive the necessary application materials after the request has been received.

Then, the heavy-duty paperwork begins. The scholarship committee may require any number of records, in addition to the completed application. They may ask for academic records, several letters of recommendation, and ACT or SAT scores. It may take several extra weeks for the institutions to receive the test scores after the student requests that they be sent.

Also, a college or university may require a personal statement from the applicant, something like a one-page autobiography, explaining some of the more important aspects of his personality. They will want to know the student's motivation for pursuing a particular field.

Many institutions want to get a feel for the type of character possessed by the students in whose futures they are investing. Since so many of these programs give large sums of money and ask nothing in return, they want to spend that money as wisely as possible.

Is a particular student really serious about becoming educated?

Is he or she going to have the strength of character and the determination to put in the hard work required to succeed?

Personal Statements Are Crucial to Success

When a personal statement is required, it should receive a great deal of attention. Time should be invested in writing and rewriting it until the student is sure it is just right. It is crucial that a teacher or guidance counselor review it and offer constructive criticism, because a student will not have the experience necessary to know exactly what he or she should write.

When a person asks some institution to which he or

she is a stranger to be forthcoming with a large sum of money, the request must be extremely persuasive!

The people whose jobs it is to select a limited number of winners from a large pool of applicants have nothing to go by except the credentials and other written information in front of them. They have no opportunity to sit down and get to know how wonderful and kind-hearted or how worthy of help each applicant may be.

They can only hope to develop some sense of each individual from what is written in this personal statement. Therefore, it behooves each applicant to try to impress the selection committee in every way possible in this statement.

When a student hands in an application packet in which there are misspelled words, basic grammatical errors, and a carelessly written personal statement, it tells the committee several things. The committee members will think the student does not take their program seriously enough to put forth his best effort, or they will think his best effort is very weak — which is even worse.

Regardless of what they think, you can be sure that applicant will be passed over in favor of someone who invested more time and effort into submitting a more professional application.

It would be a great mistake for anyone to neglect the input of a guidance counselor or teacher, when writing a personal statement. Even if a student makes straight A's in English, grammar is only one aspect of a good personal statement. It also needs to be powerful and persuasive, as well as pertinent.

When I wrote my first draft for the personal statement to send in with my medical school application, I thought I had done a good job. After all, I was a college graduate. I thought I knew what I wanted and needed to say to impress the committee.

Fortunately, I asked the pre-med counselor to read it

before I submitted it. To my surprise, he practically tore it to shreds!

I had said many things he showed me were irrelevant from the viewpoint of a selection committee. On the other hand, I had left out important things that should have been included. Furthermore, some sentences were either too wordy or too unclear.

There were numerous areas in that statement that needed to be ironed out. When the counselor gave me the paper back, it looked as if a child had taken a red pen and scribbled all over it.

I wrote that statement over and over, each time giving it to my counselor to read and critique. He sat down with me personally on several occasions and gave me great insight into things for which the committee would be looking. He showed me what they would find impressive and what would bore them or actually "turn them off."

By the time I got to what he considered the final draft, I could see a tremendous improvement. The first draft, which once had seemed "good enough," then appeared terribly inadequate. I was very grateful for the guidance and input. Also, I learned to use a thesaurus.

A *thesaurus* is a book similar to a dictionary, except that it only gives a brief definition, but is followed by a list of words with similar meanings. This enables writers to expand their vocabularies and make their writings more colorful and exciting without using the same words over and over.

In another situation, I was asked to read the personal statements of a group of black high school students applying for a job in a scientific research laboratory. This job was part of a minority program set up to expose black youth to health care careers.

These students obviously had not been coached as to the importance of having a personal statement proofread or critiqued. Most of them had numerous basic punctuation, grammatical and spelling errors.

The content and ideas of their statements were fine for high school students. However, the written expression of those ideas was very poor. If they had only taken the time to have their statements looked over by a teacher, guidance counselor, or even someone qualified to catch basic errors, most of the statements would have gone from being poor to being very good.

Furthermore, the majority of them made very careless errors which they themselves could have caught, if they had carefully proofread their own material.

This is just another of the countless instances in which intelligent black youth "miss the boat," so to speak, due to a lack of understanding about how to compete in our highly competitive society.

Regardless of one's situation, the personal statement is extremely important and deserves a great deal of attention. I cannot stress enough the importance of obtaining guidance from outside sources.

The Relationship Between Education and Employment

No one can dispute the fact that a good education is extremely important these days. The following table demonstrates the relationship between education and employment status:

Unemployment Rate (%) of Persons 25 Years Old and Older: 1992

	White	Black	Hispanic
Less than a high school graduate	10.7	15.1	12.8

| High school graduate, no college | 6.0 | 12.3 | 9.0 |
| Bachelor's degree or higher | 3.0 | 4.4 | 5.0 |

Source: U.S. Dept. of Labor, Bureau of Labor Statistics, Office of Employment and Unemployment Statistics, unpublished data.

As one can see from the above statistics, the unemployment rate decreases as the level of education increases. Not only does education decrease the chance for being unemployed, it also increases the earning potential dramatically.

Adults who did not have an opportunity to go to college or young adults who only now realize the need for more education do not have to consider their chances over with. There are numerous training programs available for adults who would like to learn a trade.

There also are evening classes available at many colleges, particularly city colleges, through which an adult can earn a college degree and still hold down a full-time job. This is not as easy as going full-time to college and, of course, it takes longer; however, it is well worth the sacrifice.

As these schools cater to adults, not teenagers, they are set up to accommodate the schedules of their students who are already employed at jobs. For example, a person who works from 9 a.m. to 5 p.m. Mondays through Fridays may sign up for evening classes. Conversely, someone who works nights can sign up for morning classes.

A person can even sign up for a combination of morning, afternoon, and evening classes, if that is necessary. These training sessions can last from a few weeks up to several years, depending on the area of study.

Someone who has trouble making ends meet can still afford to get training. Most schools offer financial assistance in the form of grants that never have to be paid back and guaranteed government loans which do.

Grants are based on financial need. Therefore, those people in the worst financial situations are favored for these awards. Loans can be set up through private organizations or through the government. The most popular is the Stafford loan that I mentioned previously.

With a Stafford loan, a person often can pay tuition and fees and perhaps have money left over to help with transportation and other expenses. The maximum amount for which a person is approved varies according to multiple factors, such as the school's tuition, the person's income, number of dependents, living expenses, and so forth.

Regardless of the situation, most people who do not make a great deal of money can qualify for these government loans. The government pays the interest as long as the person is enrolled in school at least half time.

Furthermore, no loan payments are due until six months after the person finishes his training program. Ordinarily, this allows plenty of time to get a good paying job in his chosen field. Even when monthly payments do start, usually they are low.

In the event a graduate has a problem finding a job, he can make arrangements for an additional grace period during which time he does not have to make his usual monthly payments.

Some people would argue that they do not want to get into debt. However, consider the fact that a person can go from earning minimum wage working like a dog to making significantly more than that while doing much more interesting, intellectually stimulating, and emotionally rewarding work. In that light, that small monthly payment for a few years becomes insignificant.

A person can easily increase his yearly salary by much more than the entire loan in the first year after training is completed.

It's Never Too Late for an Education

There are many well-paying fields that do not require a four-year college degree, as well. To get started, look in the yellow pages under schools or universities. Call a variety of them and request brochures on their programs and on the financial assistance available.

Furthermore, much of the same information previously presented for teenagers who want to get an education is just as applicable to adults. For instance, *The College Blue Book* provides a tremendous amount of information for anyone seeking financial assistance to pay for training.

Age should never be a factor when it comes to getting an education.

It does not matter how old an individual is when he decides to explore and cultivate his true potential. I began medical school training when I was several years older than most of my classmates.

Furthermore, there were some other students in my class who were in their forties, married, and rearing several children. At the same time, they were studying night and day to become physicians.

Going back to school can be very challenging, but it can also be even more rewarding. Even those who never graduated from high school can study for the high school equivalency exam around their own schedules and take the test when they are ready.

For these individuals, phoning the local department of education would be a good place to start. However, for those not so inclined, there still are a variety of training programs that do not even require a high school diploma. Again, the yellow pages would be a great place to start learning about the programs available in any given area.

There is a field out there to suit every personality type.

Learning a trade only requires a strong desire, motivation, dedication, and the right information to get started.

Summary

African-Americans are every bit as brilliant and capable as any other race of people. Unfortunately, for a wide variety of reasons (most of which we have discussed in this book), as a whole the race lags significantly behind most other races in terms of level of educational achievement, and consequently, income and self-esteem.

There are many avenues available for both youth and adults to obtain a challenging and rewarding education. However, many times great obstacles, ranging from lack of self-confidence to lack of appropriate information, must be overcome prior to an individual truly realizing his God-given potential for growth and success.

In order to prevent falling further and further behind as this highly advanced society continues to move forward, the African-American mind must be rejuvenated.

Little children's minds must be strengthened and encouraged in order for their futures to be bright.

Millions of high school dropouts must reconsider their career options and take a positive step forward.

Information about a wide variety of educational programs, as well as financial assistance, needs to be spread throughout the black community. People of all ages stand to benefit tremendously from this information. Individuals who are well-informed should advertise this information to the best of their ability.

If we work together to encourage one another and build each other up, putting aside all the petty envying and strife that hold us back as a people, we can once again realize our true intellectual potential demonstrated by our

African ancestors, the ancient Egyptians, who revolutionized the fields of math and science with their mind-boggling
pyramids.

Throughout the years, we have not lost any of our
God-given intelligence, just our love and respect for one
another and our pride in ourselves and our race. However,
if we can recapture these vital elements of success, there will
be no limit to what we can accomplish for our race and for
all mankind.

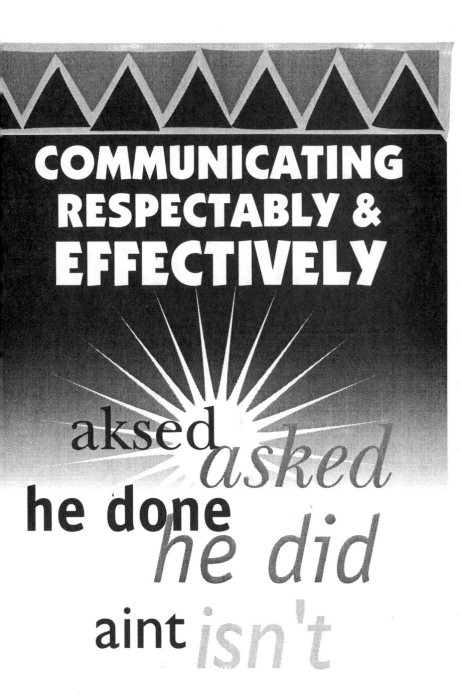

COMMUNICATING RESPECTABLY & EFFECTIVELY

aksed
asked

he done
he did

aint
isn't

Good Grammar Is Not a "White" Standard

by A. Maria Newsome, M.D.

Very few Americans today of any color use perfect grammar. However, there is a certain level of competency considered necessary to be comprehensible even by persons of relatively low intelligence. The general academic standard in America is lower than that of the British Commonwealth countries, for example, and has declined for most of this century.

Recently, a journalism professor at a major Christian university had to add a basic English course to the requirements for a degree. Too many high school students were entering college without being able to spell basic words, without a knowledge of basic grammar, and not being able to read fluently much above what used to be considered a sixth-grade level.

It is important to know and speak English correctly because at this point it is an international language. Just as Greek was nearly everyone's "second" language in the time of Jesus, so English is — worldwide — today. The same fundamental rules of grammar apply throughout the world wherever people speak English.

Nelson Mandela, head of the African National Congress (ANC) of South Africa, and Raisa Gorbachev, former "first lady" of the Soviet Union, use the same internationally accepted rules of English usage. Both speak beautiful English, better than most Americans, white or black!

However, many white children have the advantage of growing up in a society in which the same English is reinforced at home and at school. There is little chance for confusion when your parents teach you the same English that your teachers teach.

On the other hand, there are some pockets remaining, particularly in the Southern Appalachians, where white children have what amounts to their own version of English. When these mountain "throwbacks" to Elizabethan-English days enter public schools, they have to almost learn to speak all over again or continue to sound illiterate. Some very famous country music stars fall into this category.

Many black Americans have a very serious, almost self-destructive, blind spot where language is concerned. Like the Appalachian whites, blacks have developed their own form of English that sometimes is called "street talk" and sometimes "just the way blacks talk." However, if we want to compete in the marketplace and credibly hold our own within society, we must learn to give up our comfortable, traditional "black" language and learn proper English.

Good grammar and speech is not "a white standard" but a worldwide standard in any nation, among all races and colors.

Unfortunately, black grammar has come to be an extremely sensitive subject, one which causes a lot of nostrils to "flare." However, *it desperately needs to be addressed!* Actually, poor grammar is so much a part of black culture that many people — white *and* black — not only accept substandard English from blacks but expect it.

What is even worse is that many blacks *cling* to inferior English as a mark of black identity. They seem to fear that learning to speak properly will turn them into the proverbial "oreo." Compare the errors in the following letters:

Dear Joyce,

What's going on *gurl* (girl)? Nothing much is happening on the home front. Mom and Dad are doing fine and send *there* (their) love. Little *tommy* (Tommy) finally got a summer job working as a waiter. Can you believe it? He's growing up so *quikly* (quickly). Our little brother spends half his money on himself, but gives the other half to the folks. Isn't that sweet?

Do you *remeber* (remember) Cheryl from school? Well, she is getting *married* (married) next month, and I'm going to be a bridesmaid. She must have *sint* (sent) an invitation to everyone in the county. You know she doesn't have any sense!

How's life in the big city? I'll be coming to visit as soon as I get my *vacashun* (vacation) scheduled. When are you going to get your *phon* (phone) hooked up? I'm getting tired of having to *rite* (write) all of the time.

Well, I just wanted to drop a line to say *helo* (hello). I need to start getting *redy* (ready) to go to work. Be sweet.

Love,

Inger

Dear Joyce,

What's going on, girl? Nothing much *be* (is) happening on the home front. Mom and Dad are doing fine and send *they* (their) love. Little Tommy finally got a summer job. He *work* (works, or "is working") as a waiter at Cooper's. Can you believe it? Our little brother has *got* (has) a job. *He* (is) growing up so quickly. He *spend* (spends) half his money on *hisself* (himself) and *give* (gives) the rest to the folks. Isn't that sweet?

Do you remember Cheryl from high school? Well, *she* (is) getting married next month, and I'm going to be a bridesmaid. She must have sent an invitation to everyone in the county. You know she *aint got no* (has no, or hasn't any) sense!

How's life in the big city? I'll be coming to visit as soon as I get my vacation time scheduled. When are you going to get your phone hooked up? I'm tired of writing all the time.

Well, I just wanted to drop a line to say hello. I need to start getting ready to go to work. Be sweet.

Love,

Inger

The first letter has a number of spelling errors, but the errors in the second letter are even more basic. People learn to speak before they learn how to write. They involve breaking common rules of grammar. Sadly, many blacks would not only think the second letter was all right but become very angry if you tried to change their way of speaking.

Anyone Can Learn Proper Speech: Ask Eliza Doolittle

Eliza Doolittle is the heroine of George Bernard Shaw's classic book, *Pygmalion*. Made into an Oscar-winning movie in 1938, it was remade as a Broadway musical with Julie Andrews in 1956 and as a Hollywood musical in 1964 with Audrey Hepburn as "Eliza." You may know it better by its Broadway and movie title, *My Fair Lady*.

The plot of book, play, and film is centered around a girl who sold flowers on the street and spoke very improper "Cockney" English. On a dare, she was transformed by

Professor Higgins (played in the play and film by Rex Harrison) into someone who could take her place among the "upper crust" of British society.

Of course, her transformation involved manners and the right clothes, but the main focus of the change was her speech patterns and grammatical usage.

As Higgins is strolling along the market streets of London's Soho District with a famous scholar of the dialects of India, his ear is afflicted with the sounds of "the King's English" being butchered right and left.

He says of Eliza, "Look at her, a prisoner of the gutter, condemned by every syllable she utters. By rights, she should be taken out and hanged for the cold-blooded murder of the English tongue."

In one of the popular, award-winning Lerner and Loewe songs in the musical, Higgins goes on to comment: "Why can't the English teach their children how to speak? Norwegians learn Norwegian. The Greeks are taught their Greek. In France, every Frenchman knows his language from A to Z... The Arabians learn Arabian with the speed of summer lightning. And Hebrews learn it backwards, which is absolutely frightening! (Hebrew is written from right to left instead of left to right as we do.)

"Oh, why can't the English," Higgins sings, "why can't the English learn to speak?"

The "draggle-tailed guttersnipe" listens to Higgins boast of being able to turn her into a highly respectable, sophisticated woman and begins to dream of a better job with the consequences of a warm apartment, nice furniture and clothes, "and lots and lots of chocolates."

The video is available for home viewing and is well-worth seeing. The plot may sound farfetched, but in reality, it is not. "Class" is not a matter of birth nor of money, but of how one carries oneself.

This movie would be profitable for blacks to see because it shows graphically that the issue of speaking one's native language poorly or well is a dividing line to separate classes — not races — all over the world.

Proper use of language is *not* merely another racial problem between American whites and blacks. Who can forget Hollywood's stereotypical "dumb-blonde" characters? Those ladies are simply gorgeous to look at, beautifully dressed, and wore expensive jewelry. Yet the moment they opened their mouths, all chance of gaining respect went out the window.

Clothes, jewelry, and hair-do cannot offset one's speech patterns, which mean the difference between success and failure, being respected and recognized and being slighted. Clothes do not "make the man," they simply create a facade for the real person who is exposed as soon as he or she speaks.

As African-Americans, we must learn to look at the whole picture and not focus only on our cultural biases. To do so will seriously impede our progress as a race. To take our rightful place in society, we must be like the marketing experts and analyze the "market" in order to make a place for ourselves.

Incidentally, this is not something only blacks have to do. Any person of any race has to do the same thing to be accepted as a valid and credible member of society. Many whites reared in the South must learn how to talk without the accent in order to make it in other regions and vocations.

Actually, much of what is considered a "black" accent is simply Southern. Even those blacks who moved North took the patterns of speech with them from "down home." Some people in other regions can hear a Southern white and a Northern black on the phone and not be able to tell the difference as far as accent, intonations, and speech patterns.

However, blacks have developed their own phraseology and grammatical usage that is peculiarly "black."

Despite the fact that poor grammar in the black community is a reflection of habit, learned patterns from parents, grandparents, or other family members, and the infiltration of street talk, too many people take black speech as an indication of a lower intelligence quotient.

Inferior English Is a Mark of Oppression, Not a Mark of "Black Identity"

Without a doubt, there is a great deal of truth to the argument that speaking English correctly has not been part of our black heritage. However, that does not mean we cannot now change as Eliza Doolittle did.

Taking a disadvantage forced on us by oppressors in the past centuries and turning it into a symbol of black pride is like a kidnapping victim perversely but proudly embracing derogative habits forced on her by her kidnapper.

The first representatives of the black race forcibly brought to these shores did not learn to speak English using poor grammar by choice. After the trauma of being transported in the slave ships that were basically "hell-holes" of misery and disease, they were forced to stand in markets for sale like cattle. Everyone had to be brainwashed in order for slavery to succeed.

Anything which would have demonstrated that Africans were simply human beings of a different color, complete with tremendous intellect and compassion, would have weakened the moral support many whites gave to slavery. As long as blacks were considered sub-human, ignorant, and a much-inferior race, enslaving them to wait on whites and other races was justified.

Also, if slaves had been given reasons to develop higher self-esteem, there would have been more open rebellion, whites thought. Therefore, slaves were not allowed to better themselves or, usually, to become educated enough to even read or do simple sums, as we saw in the section on Education. Their natural, God-given wit had to be hidden.

Intelligent blacks were a tremendous threat to the status quo and, if perceived as such, usually were killed or greatly persecuted.

Also, slaves learned the language of their masters but not usually *from* the masters. Instead, they learned the hard way from uneducated overseers and plantation managers, who themselves often were illiterate and not versed in the use of good grammar or speech.

African-Americans had no choice in how they learned the new language of their oppressors, having been denied self-respect and dignity in the name of "white supremacy."

With no opportunity for a formal education, being forced to speak in a kind of "code" in order not to be understood by the masters, and having to learn from uneducated teachers, it was after the Civil War before blacks began to get any kind of proper education.

Even after the war, the evils of racism — oppression, enforced poverty, segregation, death threats, and so forth — kept blacks from obtaining a quality education, one equal to whites. Blacks were still expected to accept a very lowly status in life. Countless obstacles were placed in the way of success and independence.

Laws, written and unwritten, made perimeters beyond which they could not go. I have seen an old filmstrip, a documentary, that is horrifying in its depiction of matter of fact brutality. A middle-aged white man talked to the interviewer of the town's regular Sunday social gathering. He explained that part of the weekly program was to "kill a nigger."

If they could not find one in the local jail, they just caught a black person walking up the street. In the background of this interview, you can see the latest victim dangling from a tree branch, burned beyond recognition. This kind of behavior not only created tragic and lasting trauma among blacks, but had a dehumanizing effect on the whites involved. As a matter of fact, white children were playing around the area, and adults were socializing.

To them, it was a good "down home" shindig with the added attraction of all the thrills and chills of a human sacrifice. They called blacks "animals" and "savages" all the while they were being entertained by the screams of those they tortured and murdered. More than a thousand lynchings were carried out, and for decades no white person was convicted of these inhumane and gruesome murders.

The entire judicial system, including politicians, sheriffs, judges, and juries, worked together to terrorize blacks and deprive them of basic human rights. Many whites who were not depraved enough to enjoy the torturing and murdering still fought tirelessly to keep blacks poor, ignorant, submissive, and out of sight.

Blacks lived in constant fear. They had to remain humble and simple or risk being murdered. However, many refused to accept the humiliating existence that goes with being a "downtrodden" race. Those who fought underground and out in the open risking their lives believed in the integrity of their race.They knew blacks were as beautiful and intelligent as members of any other race.

The point is that, throughout the history of blacks in America, they have not had the same educational resources for learning as whites.This lack, plus the numerous negative psychological and social factors to which blacks were and are exposed have combined to hinder African-Americans from becoming a valued and integral part of American society.

In Example Versus Tradition, Tradition Wins

Because blacks were not accepted into mainstream America until recently, most of our ancestors were not exposed to the requirements for success in this society. The majority of our parents and grandparents never learned all of the basic skills that are crucial to earning respect and achieving success in America.

This lack of experience in the marketplaces of America, coupled with the lack of quality education, created a very wide disparity between the insight that whites could pass on to their children and that which blacks could pass on to theirs.

Not having been traditionally part of mainstream America, our people have not been aware of the importance of good communication skills. Consequently, those skills have not been stressed in our homes and communities as they should have been for our children to be truly "integrated" into American society.

"Black" English is still in widespread use, and as a result, a large number of highly intelligent black Americans are unable to secure good jobs and obtain otherwise deserved recognition. They are not accustomed to communicating on a level that commands respect in our highly advanced society. This is a long-term, far-reaching successful outcome of the conspiracy against blacks that the most diligent racists could not have foreseen.

Schools *are* integrated now, so black and white children go to school together. They get the same education. Teachers in public schools now not only teach proper English but use it in front of students.

Furthermore, television is "the great leveler." On the majority of the shows until recently, even Southern whites were either the villains or the "comic relief" *simply because of the way they spoke, the phrases they used, and the drawling accent.*

In other words, use of regular, non-accented, good grammatical English is portrayed as desirable every day in front of our black children. Yet most of them still talk like our parents and grandparents did. Why?

To make the point even clearer, Asians and other foreigners come to this country and learn English as a second or even third language. Many of them speak better than blacks or whites who only know one language. Many of these people work their way quickly to the top and hold positions in which they can hire or not hire blacks. Why?

The answer is that when it comes to *right example*, particularly after a child reaches school age, versus *tradition example* — tradition wins. Most foreigners are accustomed to speaking properly in their native languages, so they learn to speak a new language properly. Many black parents today cling to traditional patterns of speech, making the wrong kind of language example for their children.

Just because Bill Cosby has shown a different side of the black experience does not mean that has been enough to strengthen positive images of blacks in the minds of Americans. Yes, this is the "Cosby generation," but it also is the generation of skyrocketing dropout rates among black youth.

It is urgent that we realize how our "stereotyped" speech patterns play into the hands of racists, continuing to give the impression that we are of an inferior intelligence simply because we cannot communicate in good English. As a result of the deception that blacks are inferior to whites, many people of other races genuinely believe that we are not intelligent.

Poor grammar sends a resounding negative message to the world when American blacks give the impression of being incapable of learning a skill that other races learn at a young age.

Most television shows, books, and newspapers generally follow standard rules of grammar, making people who speak poor English appear even more "dense." Generally speaking, all Americans of whatever race are "television junkies." So how is it that correct English can be poured into their heads for hours every day and evening, yet many view-

ers never catch on that their own speech patterns and grammatical skills are grossly different than the norm?

The answer lies in the home environment. As long as
parents accept poor grammatical skills in themselves, they
will continue to send mixed messages to their children. On
the one hand, they tell their children that education is of
primary importance, yet they do not talk at home as the child
is being taught to speak at school.

This places the child in a difficult position. Does he
seemingly repudiate his family, or does he ignore what he
learns and hears as good English and follow tradition? Quite
a dilemma, is it not?

In my own neighborhood growing up, it was not
socially acceptable for a black person to speak English
correctly. Blacks who did were quickly "converted" or risked
being ostracized and labeled as "white."

There was a tremendous amount of peer pressure to
use ungrammatical English. As a matter of fact, it was practically a prerequisite to being accepted in any "cool" social
circles. Only "nerdy" people and "wannabes" were said to
use good grammar.

Even black adults are pressured by this misplaced pride
in "black English" and forced to accept this false standard
or not be accepted by their peers. A sorority sister of mine,
who majored in communications at a predominantly black,
Southern college, told me that she was verbally attacked by
another communications major for "being so articulate."

After that, she found herself consciously trying to use
poor English in order "to fit in."

Preaching What I Practice: Some Real Life Examples

After graduating from college and doing some work
toward a Master's Degree, I planned to train to become a
doctor. There were still a great many things about English

that puzzled me. I will grant you that language experts say English is one of the hardest languages to learn. So I went to a local bookstore and bought several books and workbooks on basic English grammar.

My last course in grammar had been seven years before. In most colleges, grammar is considered such a basic skill that it is not included in the curriculum. Personally, I became dumbfounded at my own ignorance. I practically failed an advanced high school English practice test in one of the workbooks!

There were many principles which I had long since forgotten and others I am not sure I ever knew. Those books helped me tremendously, and ever since, I have tried to "preach" to others in the black community — particularly young people — these truths that I practice for myself. (I will share a list of things that helped me improve my own language skills later in this section.)

Recently, I worked with a girls' club project in a housing development in Memphis, Tennessee, where I met many beautiful, brilliant young black girls between the ages of nine and eleven. Many of them could easily handle the "hard" classes in math and science, but their basic English skills were very poor. Most of their sentences had no verbs or the wrong verbs, far below the level one would expect from children half their age.

The faculty advisor for the club told me that she actually left the center almost in tears at times because the girls' grammar was so awful. To the average American, these extremely smart girls would have appeared extremely dumb because of the way they talked.

Along with sessions on drug education and pregnancy prevention, the advisor and I tried to slip in English word games and talks about the importance of good communication skills. However, the bad grammar was so ingrained that what we tried to do was almost useless. The girls did not know how to correct mistakes when they were pointed out.

Most of them saw no reason to speak correctly. No one around them did, and in the few hours we had each month, it was not possible to change the speech habits of their entire lives. It is very sad that no matter how often these girls make the honor rolls or receive various recognitions and achievement awards, the future available employment market for them will in no way reflect their true intellectual potential.

Knowing they are smart, yet continually being turned down for good jobs will reinforce the belief that racism has kept them down. The tragic thing is that many times defeat will have come out of their own mouths and have nothing to do with racism.

During my first year of medical school, I had the opportunity to talk with approximately 100 high school and college students wanting to pursue a career in the health care field. This school had a reputation for discriminating against black applicants, and this program was designed to increase the number of qualified black applicants to health-care colleges.

This was a preprofessional program set up to expose blacks to medicine, pharmacy, and other health-related careers. There were more black students in that one program than in the entire university. Consequently, making a good impression was of the utmost importance. Students were housed without charge, got free meals, and spending money twice a month.

By living in the dorm and eating in the cafeteria, I was able to get to know some of the students. Overall, their use of English was extremely distressing to me, considering that this group was "the cream of the crop" of young black students in Tennessee, having been selected from many black young people statewide.

Other black students enrolled at the university agreed with me that these intelligent young people were giving a false impression of themselves. After talking with various professors and teachers in the program, the black man in charge set up a meeting for me to talk to the entire group about the importance of communications skills.

Our efforts were undercut, however, by one black English professor who had tremendous "black pride," evidenced by her wearing African attire from head to toe. She vehemently denied that the students spoke English poorly and verbally attacked me for suggesting such a thing. In reality, when the students were in her presence, they probably did speak better English than they used in the cafeterias.

Somehow the word got around about my upcoming talk. Despite realizing that I would be speaking to a hostile audience prepared to give me a hard time because of misunderstanding my motives, I felt compelled to go ahead. I knew they literally had no idea of the bad impression their speech was giving.

Remembering something my mother said to me when I was a difficult teenager helped me. She said that, when you truly care for someone, you do what is best for that person whether or not it causes him or her to like you. Because I genuinely cared about these students, it was my responsibility to share what I had learned, having had more opportunities than most blacks.

The talk was not very well received, and the discussion became very heated at times. A few thanked me afterwards, but the general consensus was the same two fallacies that have helped to hold blacks back in society: *Grammar is not very important in the overall scheme of things, and anyway, using poor grammar is an important part of being black.*

I had to hope that, after running into several employment walls, some might perhaps consider whether I had been right and upgrade their communication skills.

In fact, the most vocal opponent became a good friend the next year and was very apologetic for his attitude during that discussion.

Good Grammar Will Not Erase Racism, But It Will Help Us Economically

The blatant rejection of standard English does nothing to benefit blacks. Instead, it does a great deal to stunt our economic growth. This is a capitalistic society where only the strong succeed. If a person takes no pride in his language, why would an employer believe he would take pride in his work? No firm can afford to present a negative image to the public.

It would be unrealistic to expect that using better English will wipe out racism. However, it is equally unrealistic to expect that employers and co-workers will respect intelligence and abilities if we fail the most important skill taught to even preschool children — how to talk properly.

I am not saying that race is never a factor in whether one gets hired or not, but we should look at blacks who do have great jobs and see why they succeeded when others failed. Almost invariably, you will find that those with the best careers have good communication skills.

Competitiveness is the key to success, and for every well-paying job, there usually are many applicants. Why deliberately give yourself a handicap? We should never settle for less than the best from ourselves.

Our struggle for equality is far from over, although it is not usually fought on the streets now. From this point on, the struggle will require determination, pride in the right things, humility to know that we must improve ourselves in order to compete economically, and insight.

If our ancestors who suffered and died for black equality and black excellence could see how complacent we have become as a race, they would be extremely disappointed in us. They were strong and proud to be black, not willing to take inferior jobs and serve whites who were neither better nor smarter than they. However, they had no choice; we do, because they laid their lives on the line for future generations of blacks.

For anyone, black or white, to make grave grammatical errors and think no one notices or cares is extremely unrealistic. You can be liked and even loved on the basis of your personality, but you cannot be respected if you are unprofessional in any way.

The power of persuasion is a powerful tool. With it Martin Luther King, Jr. led blacks through the Civil Rights era, culminating what began with the Emancipation Proclamation. If he had spoken mostly "black English," would he even have gained a hearing, much less the respect of whites and blacks alike?

Some argue that adopting standard English would be "selling out." However, the only people we would be selling out are the massive numbers of racists responsible for creating this gap in education and communication from the day the first slave boat landed up to the present. It is closed-minded and arrogant for anyone of any race to refuse to better himself and grow.

Real Life Examples

Case One — A close black friend on the admissions committee of a large medical school told me of two recent cases of extremely intelligent black applicants who were not accepted because of their very poor basic language skills.

A great irony is that one of these students graduated at the top of her class from the university where the professor who came against my remarks so strongly teaches English. The sad thing is that, probably, there are many more such examples out there.

A second terrible irony is that, although both these students made top grades in the "difficult" classes of physics, chemistry, and calculus, they were passed over for medical careers because they had not mastered an elementary skill most Americans are exposed to before they even begin kindergarten.

The other three interviewers agreed with my friend on refusing these two applicants. By the way, this friend is a perfect example of the fact that one does not have to have great advantages to develop good communications skills. She grew up in a small country town where substandard English was a way of life.

Realizing early that she would have to be able to communicate on a respectable level to get ahead in life, she made learning correct grammar a priority. She patterned her speech after those she heard on television and sought extra coaching from her teachers, as well as from reading books.

At the same point in time, other blacks with lower admission test scores than the two students in question *were* admitted. Becoming a physician requires a highly professional demeanor that commands respect and credibility from patients and colleagues, as well as an intelligence level high enough to pass medical school.

Case Two — A former classmate now is a government attorney. After she was hired, a co-worker told her that two other blacks had applied for the job ahead of her. They were not hired because their grammar was very poor. These were attorneys who, you would think, must know that lawyers must speak well. Yet poor grammar had become such a habit that it caused them to slip up when they needed to make a crucial impression.

Case Three — While working my way through college, I had a job in Atlanta that required hiring and training new employees for the telemarketing division of a new business. As badly as people were needed by the company, I could not hire many of the blacks who applied. Their basic grammar skills were so poor they could not possibly have done well over the phone.

They were well-dressed and enthusiastic, and the job did not require great abilities. The only real skill required — to be able to converse intelligently and persuasively — was not possible for them with their low language skills.

Sadly enough, the two young ladies with the worst grammar seemed to be the most in need of jobs.

I went ahead and hired them, planning to work with them individually and help them improve their conversational abilities. However, during a monitoring session, one girl's approach was so ungrammatical that the prospective customer said, "You've got to be kidding!"

The boss demanded that I fire her. Fortunately, both employees quit before I could do so. This situation had no racism involved. In fact, I was promoted over a white employee with seniority for the same reason: She had poor communication skills. Her English was only borderline correct.

I have always regretted not being frank with the black applicants as to why I could not hire them, because they probably continued to lose jobs through making bad impressions. At that time, however, I was still young and inexperienced enough to be concerned about *their* becoming offended or even angry.

Case Four — The end result of being turned down for job after job or promotion after promotion and not knowing exactly why can be tragic. I once had a patient who was in the psychiatric ward of a hospital for suicidal depression because he could not support his children.

He had injured his back earlier and was not able to do manual labor. He obviously had tried very hard to get a desk job, but he presented himself very poorly, making basic grammatical errors in almost every sentence and several in some sentences.

Because of his dangerous condition, I could not afford to worry about "stepping on toes," so I explained why he might be having doors slammed in his face. I also assured him that poor grammar was simply a habit and no reflection of one's intelligence. Working with him to correct this habit, I encouraged him to talk more slowly and think out what he wanted to say in order to break the thought patterns of bad grammar.

In spite of that, "he be, she been done, I ain't got no, he think," and other such errors came out of his mouth almost as frequently as before. When I asked him to go back and correct what he had said wrong, most of the time he could not. He simply did not know the correct way to speak.

This grown man in his late thirties had lost the ability to distinguish between correct and incorrect grammar through the longstanding habit of incorrect usage. Consequently, he had lost the ability to demonstrate his true intellectual potential to others.

The Emperor's New Clothes

Hollywood quite often perpetuates the stereotype of blacks who massacre the English language. Some of these scripts are even written by blacks!

The reason for them is that most script writers try to develop characters to which the public can relate. The underlying assumption is that most blacks are illiterate. The sad reality is that a high percentage of American blacks not only use poor grammar but see no problem with it!

There are countless jokes involving black English in wide circulation, and it is not always whites laughing at blacks. Many blacks laugh as well.

It reminds me of the old tale, "The Emperor's New Clothes." A couple of con men had convinced an emperor that the invisible clothes they made for him were more beautiful than any he already had.

Paying the scoundrels for the "clothes," the emperor began walking around naked. No one was willing to tell him the true state of things for fear he would be angry or for fear they would be ostracized for not pretending like everyone else that he was wearing clothes. One little boy finally had the courage to tell the emperor there were no clothes, and he actually was naked.

Concerning the communications skills of a high percentage of African-Americans, someone needs to stand up and shout, "The Emperor is naked!"

Strategies for Improvement

by A. Maria Newsome, M.D.

I used the following strategies to learn better communication, and I recommend them to others also in search of methods of improving their language skills.

1. *Purchase a book on English grammar.* I strongly recommend buying this as a beginning. Many of them are not expensive, perhaps less than $10, and can be found in any bookstore.

2. *Make personal notes.* While reading the morning newspaper or a good book, use a colored pencil or ink pen to underline words and groups of words that are used differently than you would have phrased them.

Pay special attention to which verb conjugation is used with different subjects and in different time frames. Jot these things down in a small notebook kept handy just for this purpose. By reviewing these notes from time to time, standard English may be learned and reinforced with modest effort.

3. *Form the habit of correcting yourself when you hear yourself speaking incorrectly.* This will train your ear to listen for bad grammar in your own speech as well as in that of others.

4. *Make it a point to pronounce words as clearly as possible.* You might tape yourself talking sometimes and play it back

to see how you sound. Pay attention to the way difficult words are pronounced on television or news shows.

5. *Don't be afraid to ask for other people's opinions about the way you speak.* I have learned a lot by doing so. Very few people will come right out and tell you that you speak poorly, so ask those you respect for their own language skills to tell you where you need to improve.

Following is a miniature lesson in grammar that some may find helpful. Obviously, this does not cover all the possible grammatical errors. However, these are the ones which I hear blacks use most often. In addition, I have included similar errors that are not in widespread use to serve as a comparison in order to bring home how awkward "black English" sounds to others.

By viewing comparable errors and realizing how peculiar they sound, it makes it easier to realize how unintelligent some of these more common errors sound to others.

Error	Explanation	Comparable Error
Theyself	Non-existent word Correct words are: themselves, himself	**Youself**
I be, you be	There are very limited situations in which "be" can be used this way. "If that be true" is correct, but "She be playing too much," is not. It is safer to avoid using "be" as a verb unless you understand this rule of grammar.	**You am, I are**

They house, **They clothes**	"They" is a pronoun used for more than one person, while "their" indicates possession.	**He house** **She clothes**
	These two words are not used interchangeably.	
You was **We was** **They was**	The correct usage is: I was they were you were we were it/he/she was	**I were standing there.** **It were given to me.**
I, you done he/she/it done we or they done	Done needs a helping verb. "I *have* done it," or She *has* done it" are correct. Alternatively, the intended meaning of the sentence may simply require changing *done* to *did* in certain situations.	**I gone somewhere.** **She known that for a long time.**
She think **He need** **She know**	Basic subject-verb conjugation is one of the first skills taught in school because it is so important. *He* knows/*He* needs, etc. *She* knows/*She* needs, etc. *It* knows/*It* needs, etc. They know, they need, etc. You know, you need, etc. This is the same pattern used for most simple verbs in the English language. Without mastering this pattern, a person is unlikely to impress anyone with his or her communication skills.	**I thinks I'll go.** **We knows better.**

She do/don't   This is another striking error in   **I does it.**
He do/don't   basic subject-verb agreement.   **You does it.**
                     Correct usage is I do, you do,
                     he/it does, we do, they do.
                     Obviously, as "don't" is a
                     contraction for *do not*, and
                     one cannot say "He/she/it
                     do not," then one cannot say
                     "He/she/it don't" either.
                     One should say, "He/she/it
                     does not" or "doesn't."

Ain't   *Ain't* is always wrong, no exceptions!

We don't have   This is called a "double negative." When
no....   two negative words are used together, they
                     cancel each other out and change the intended
                     meaning completely. Similarly, multiplying
                     a negative number by a negative number gives
                     a positive number. *Don't* means "do not," and
                     no means "no." To say that you *don't have no*
                     something actually says you *do not have no*
                     whatever it is, which means that you *do* have
                     some. "I don't have *no* money," means you do
                     have some money.

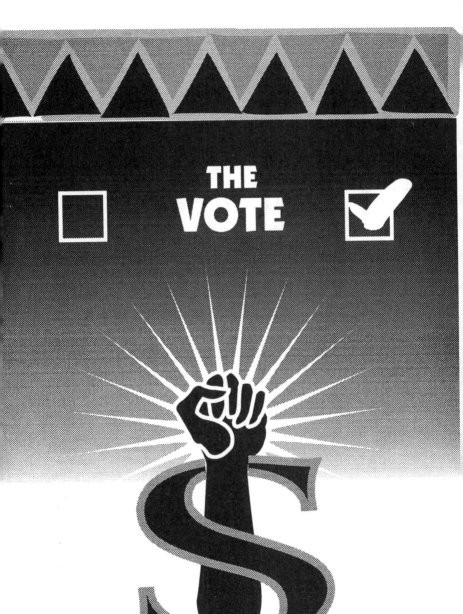

Institutionalizing a Political and Economic Empowerment Agenda

by Cleo Washington, Attorney at Law,
City Councilman

[Author's Note: This chapter examines the compelling necessity for African-Americans to develop a comprehensive political and economic empowerment agenda by the year 2000 as a method for *Bridging the Gap*. It is the opinion of the author that clergy, elected officials, educators, and entrepreneurs must collaborate to institutionalize the agenda.]

History Behind the Voting Rights Act:

"The right of citizens of the United States to *vote* shall not be denied or abridged on account of race . . . ."

— Amendment XV of the U. S. Constitution
Ratified February 3, 1870

Generations-long heinous race relations in many southern states became the impetus in the 60s for civil rights organizations to pursue federal legislation to terminate the perpetual discrimination against minorities in voting.

Alabama, a state where elected officials were known for their inhospitable view towards African-Americans, was one of several states that literally became a battlefield for civil rights advocates in the 1950s and 1960s.

In early 1963, four African-American children were killed when a bomb exploded in their Birmingham church. The resulting national media coverage helped create nationwide outrage, which ultimately provided the stimulus for passage of the 1964 Civil Rights Act.

This brutal bombing served as a catalyst for mobilizing many Alabama civil rights proponents to engage in a national voter registration campaign. By January, 1965, several organizations were engaging in voting registration drives, including the Selma, Alabama, Southern Christian Leadership Conference (SCLC) and the National Association for the Advancement of Colored People (NAACP).

In the early Sunday morning hours of March 7, 1965, approximately 300 Selma residents, including many members of the SCLC, members of churches, civil rights workers, and black and white clergy met at the Brown African Methodist Episcopal Church (A.M.E.) to hold a prayer vigil before walking over to the Edward Pettus Bridge near downtown Selma.

The intention was to march to the state capitol in Montgomery and protest voter registration procedures. However, then Sheriff Jim Clark and several of his deputies in riot gear and with clubs and masks lined up at the middle of the bridge. Clark ordered the marchers to return to their church and neighborhoods.

When the marchers displayed a resolve to continue, the sheriff immediately motioned for his deputies to charge them. The attack was swift, unmerciful, and fatal. Many of the marchers received permanent injuries.

One of the most notable deaths was that of a white minister, the Rev. James J. Reeb. This day became known as

"Bloody Sunday," and the national media coverage shocked the conscience of America.

Two weeks later, on March 21, 1965, several thousand people showed up for the scheduled five-day march from Selma to Montgomery. At the completion of the march on March 26, the Rev. Martin Luther King, Jr. gave his now-famous "How long?" speech on the steps of the Alabama State Capitol:

> I know some of you are asking today, "How long will it take?" I come to say to you this afternoon, however difficult the moment, however frustrating the hour, it will not be long, because truth pressed to earth will rise again.
>
> How long? Not long, because no lie can live forever. How long? Not long, because you will reap what you sow. How long? Not long, because the arm of the moral universe is long, but it bends toward justice.

President Lyndon B. Johnson, a strong advocate of civil rights, was so disturbed by Sheriff Clark's actions that he immediately delivered his voting rights bill to Congress. The Voting Rights Act of 1965, 42 U.S.C. 1973, was passed on August 6, 1965, in an effort to enforce the requirement of the Fifteenth Amendment that the right to vote shall not be abridged.

This act suspended state literacy tests and other voter qualification tests that had been used in certain geographical areas, mostly throughout the South, to deny African-Americans the right to vote.

This act also permitted federal examiners to enter states and register voters where less than 50 percent of the voting age population was registered or voted in the November, 1964, election. It became obvious the clear intent of the United States Congress was to rid the country of racial discrimination in the electoral process.

The first case to test this act was *South Carolina vs. Katzenbach*, 383 U.S. 301 (1966), in which the state of South Carolina attempted to challenge the constitutionality of several provisions of the Voting Rights Act. In due time, the United States Supreme Court held that the Congress exercised legitimate authority granted to it by the Fifteenth Amendment when it enacted remedies for voting discrimination.

However, Congress realized before long that the restricted geographical limitations caused a major problem that could only be dealt with by passing an extension to the previous act.

The 1970 act lowered the minimum age of voters in both state and federal elections from twenty-one to eighteen, barred the use of literacy tests in all state and national elections, and abolished state durational residency requirements.

The Voting Rights Act again was extended in 1975 for seven years, making permanent the nationwide ban on literacy tests.

Many in the civil rights community believed that the primary contribution of the amendments was to finally allow African-Americans to reach their goal of multiracial power sharing. The most immediate anticipated result was the increased number of African-Americans elected as officials on the municipal level.

For example, the number of African-American mayors swelled from 108 in 1972 to 355 in 1995. However, the most significant developments came as a result of further Congressional action necessitated by a 1982 Supreme Court decision.

Misinterpretation of the Intent Requirement

The Carter Administration's Justice Department prodded legislatures of many southern states to comply with the

Voting Rights Act by redrawing districts in such a way as to not dilute the voting strength of minorities.

Civil rights groups had often complained that "multi-member districts" and "at-large" voting schemes operated to impair the ability of minorities to elect representatives of their choice. African-Americans dispersed in an overwhelmingly white majority district had their voting power diluted. Whereas single member districts would provide a greater opportunity to elect representatives of their choice.

The battleground issue surrounded the interpretation of Section 2 (a) of the Voting Rights Act. This section prohibits all states from imposing any voting process that would "*result* in the denial or abridgment of the right to vote of any citizen who is a member of a protected class or racial or language minorities."

Its companion section stated that there was a violation where the "totality of the circumstances" established that the political process leading to nomination or election was not open equally to participation by members of minority groups.

Opponents of the section argued that "intent" to discriminate against minority voters was required before a violation of the Act could be proven. The Supreme Court gave credence to this argument in its decision in *City of Mobile vs. Bolden,* 446 U.S. 55 (1980).

The Court's opinion held that African-American voters in Mobile were required to prove that the contested electoral practice had been adopted with the intent to discriminate against minority voters. Supporters of the Act were outraged by this decision and the nearly insurmountable burden it placed on minorities to prove intent.

They immediately lobbied Congress to restore the

results test, arguing that the Court wrongly applied the discriminatory intent requirement which had long governed equal protection violations. However, the Voting Rights Act was adopted pursuant to the Fifteenth Amendment. Discriminatory intent is irrelevant under the analysis of that amendment.

Attempting to prove the intent test would require allegations of racism against the legislative body drawing the districts, and an admission by legislators that race was the primary factor in drawing those lines. These allegations would only create more racial animosity and, of course, it would not have been in the best interests of the legislators in question to concede that, in fact, they had been attempting to dilute minority voting strength.

After lengthy floor debate, the U. S. Congress in 1982 again amended Section 2 of the Voting Rights Act to explicitly overrule the *City of Mobile* decision and the requirement for minority voters to prove discriminatory intent.

Four years later, the U. S. Supreme Court reviewed the 1982 amendments in a case originating in North Carolina. In *Thornburg vs. Gingles*, 478 U.S. 30 (1986), the Court concluded that the amendment eliminated "any requirement of establishing that the contested electoral practice was adopted or maintained with the intent to discriminate against minorities."

African-American civil rights leaders across the nation applauded this decision as a huge step toward multiracial power sharing. It was widely viewed that this decision would provide the basis for Congressional reapportionment throughout the South and ultimately aid African-American efforts to create "minority-majority" districts.

Minority Gains Resulted From Redistricting

The Congressional Black Caucus gained sixteen new

members in the 103rd Congress, sworn in during January, 1993. Thirteen were from predominately black southern districts created in this reapportionment. Thus their election was a direct result of the Voting Rights Act. The huge success of African-Americans in electing representatives of their choice and background resulted from having the act institutionalized in their respective states.

Many clergy, civic, political, and business leaders within the African-American community now realize that self-reliance is the only way in which our people will achieve economic emancipation. However, this will not come until there has been a consensus to articulate, develop, and disseminate an economic empowerment agenda in much the same way that the political agenda was institutionalized.

Blacks Need To Exercise the Power of the Vote

by A. Maria Newsome, M.D.

All adults need to get out and vote for those individuals who are willing to make some positive changes, not just for blacks, but for all Americans. Even if it is simply a matter of voting for the lesser of two evils, a person should *always* vote. Voters have a tremendous amount of power in electing those individuals who would best serve their needs.

Numerous African-Americans were murdered for trying to obtain political power for their people. All kinds of racist laws and tactics were used to prevent blacks from having this important power. Today, however, we have the right to help mold our communities and our schools, and very often, we fail to exercise this right.

We can vote in the 90s without fear of bombings or lynchings. That makes it even more of a travesty when a high percentage of blacks do not register to vote or choose not to take the time to vote, lightly regarding their rights that were won at such cost by some of our ancestors.

When a significant number of people do not take the time to vote, their opinions and needs carry no political weight. *They have no bargaining power.* We should learn about individual candidates and the issues they stand for or against. Voting in every election — local, state, or national

— should be a priority for every black person over voting age.

Even an eighty-five-year-old bedridden citizen can mail in an absentee ballot and be part of the governing process of this country.

REBUILDING THE
AFRICAN AMERICAN
COMMUNITY

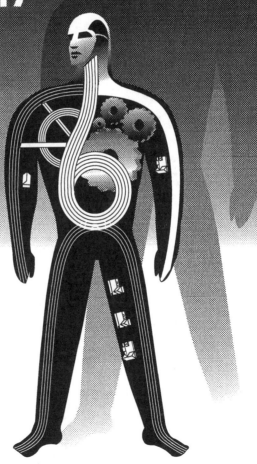

Rebuilding Our Community Is Imperative

by Lorenzo Hester: Businessman

According to Webster's Dictionary, the word *community* means:

> Fellowship (*communis*, common) — 1a) all the people living in a particular district, city, etc. . . . 2) a group of people living together as a smaller social unit within a larger one, and having interests, work, etc. in common, 3) a group of nations loosely or closely associated because of common traditions or for political or economic advantage."[1]

In most major cities across America, the inner city is where most of the undereducated, underprivileged, and socio-economically depressed people live, and the inner city is commonly defined as "the African-American community." This "community" is quickly becoming a community of have-nots robbed of valuable resources and deprived of systemic growth.

This chapter will address not only some major factors that are contributing to the degeneration of the African-American community; but, more importantly, it will address what can be done to stop this declining condition and to begin the rebuilding process. The problems with our community make a good subject for an intellectual conversation or debate in some circles.

In fact, our community problems are discussed, debated, and analyzed very intellectually from Capitol Hill in Washington, DC, to Hurt Village (a housing project) in Memphis, Tennessee. However, these many intellectual discussions and debates have produced little in terms of solutions for our community problems. Rebuilding the African-American community will take more than intellect. It will require people to acquire a sense of responsibility to one another.

There are many things the African-American community could do to strengthen itself from within. We need to take on more of the responsibility of working on our own problems. Even with the best of intentions, our leaders cannot do it all. We need to stop looking for other people to solve our problems and start looking within to solve our own problems. Looking for someone else to come into your house and clean it up for you is not the best approach.

We need to look to ourselves to find solutions. Rebuilding should start with "me." "I" can do something about my own situation; "I" should take it upon "my" shoulders to do whatever I can to make our (black America's) situation better. If it is no more than going out and encouraging someone who is less fortunate than oneself, that is a good beginning.

It is not going to do any of us any good to "sit back on our laurels" and wait for someone else to solve our problems. Who can say that "someone" will ever come? More importantly, who is to say that this "someone" is not you and me? We should all be very passionate about helping and serving our brothers, because once you start helping others, you are helping yourself as well. Life is one big circle. We are a "family," and if you help your brothers and sisters, that help undoubtedly is going to come back to you.

We are a communal people, whose shared social, economic, and religious values are the foundation of our survival. It appears that we have become disconnected from that foundation. The negative statistics relating to African-Americans in regard to disintegration of families and high crime rates appear as major contributors to discombobulating our community. However, there is a redeeming truth beyond all of the negative statistics that appear to be contributing to the upsetting of our foundation.

That *truth* is that we are a people who fear God, who are strong-spirited, and who have survived through hundreds of years of atrocities. If we are to survive these new atrocities, we must each reach within ourselves and find or renew ourselves with that truth. It has not only enabled us to survive, but it can make us towers of strength. Then we will be ready to displace those negative statistics by statistics of even more remarkable achievements.

One issue that desperately needs to be addressed is the flight of African-Americans from the inner city. No one will deny that the mass exodus of affluent blacks from predominantly black neighborhoods drains those communities of wealth, role models, and culture. The term "successful black" not only refers to those with professional status. It refers to any black person who has developed his mind and talents and is able to become a positive member of the community in spite of the obstacles he, or she, has faced.

In America's Jewish communities at the turn of the century, whenever a member of that community went to university to better himself academically, he returned to those who had supported him. He returned to contribute positively to the betterment of his community. Too often this is not the case with African-Americans. On the whole, those who have become successful seldom give back to the community in any respect. Thus, the cycle of flight from the inner cities is perpetuated. Drugs and violence often replace the social and economic wealth that successful blacks could have contributed.

Of the many areas of life affected by this pattern of flight from the inner city, one of the most pronounced is that of black children. Our children are crying out for guidance and direction, and they are looking in all the wrong places for those things. So often, children in socially and economically depressed neighborhoods have no positive role models. They see successful blacks on television, but in their own neighborhoods, there is no "supporting cast."

There are countless black children who would love to have someone give them positive guidance on where to go in life and how to get there. Not only is it worthwhile, it also is one of our duties or missions in life as responsible adults to reach out and give direction to our children; not just our own, but to the children in the community as a whole.

Through academics, athletics, or simply positive talking to our youth, we can contribute significantly to their lives. It is important to become positively involved in some aspect of a young person's life. Youth need to be led by example, not so much what they hear but what they see. Spending "quality time" with a child who needs a positive role model could make a big difference in that child's life.

Time spent encouraging and training our children undoubtedly will equip them to make better decisions. Exposing them to different aspects of society, aspects they do not often see in their inner-city neighborhoods, will have a tremendous impact on their lives. They need particularly to see African-Americans in professional positions and be encouraged thereby to set high goals for themselves. Our children would then, in turn, be in a better position to contribute positively to the community. The long-term positive effects would be immense.

There are many volunteer organizations — such as Boys

Club, Big Brothers/Sisters, Urban League, churches, and other agencies which offer opportunities for positive direct involvement in the lives of our children. Also, if you want to help but do not want to join an organization, the public schools need tutors. Another alternative is to form an inner-city sports minor league. Sports is an excellent way to reach out and get involved in the positive development of our children.

An alternative to personal involvement is donating financial support to local volunteer agencies. Help those who *are* helping. There are many other ways to participate. The important thing is to do something positive. An adult willing to make a commitment to help is the key ingredient for developing positive results in a child's life. There is an overwhelming need for successful blacks who have fled the inner cities to return and help rebuild the community by *bridging the gap* for a better tomorrow through helping our children today.

Furthermore, if our children are to be bridges spanning the gaps between today's mediocrity and tomorrow's great possibilities, then those "bridges" need strong "support pillars." It appears that our black women are doing a tremendous job in supporting this connecting effort with relatively little help from black men. The physical and emotional strength of our men is needed by our women. Together, we can forge great and mighty pillars to support our children as they bridge these gaps.

We ask those brothers who are not helping these questions: Where are you? Why are you not helping? Is it because you are lost and confused as to who you are?

I believe many black men *are* confused as to who they are, and not only confused, but angry about not knowing, about not having a connection to their heritage. The result of this disorientation has caused many to stray from family, moral values, and self-dignity, searching in many unproductive places for answers as to who they really are. This wandering and wondering has left them in such places as jail, or even the grave.

Two Perspectives of the African-American Man

Let us look at two perspectives of the African-American man: Where he is and who he is.

Where *is* the African-American man?

Of the estimated 42 million African-Americans who live in the United States, some 20 million are males. According to recent statistics from the Bureau of Justice, more than one million of them are under correctional supervision.[2] There are more African-American men locked in prisons than made the recent "Washington March." The bureau reported that, in 1993, there were 16,962 murders committed in this country. Of those, African-American men were responsible for 56 percent (9,613). Homicide is second to AIDS in killing our young black males.

A Christian Broadcasting Network (CBN) Fact Sheet in late 1995 reported that "one of every three black males [aged] 15-35 is in prison."[3] There are more young black men in prison than in colleges and universities! These are only a few of the negative statistics reflecting where the African-American male is today. One conclusion to be drawn from these statistics is that *brothers cannot vote or have positive impact on our community if they are in jail or dead.*

Who is the African-American man?

The African-American man is from a race that endured and survived hundreds of years of atrocities, slavery, and "Jim-Crowism." He is a sold-out, bought-out, turned-out, hung-up, burned-up, shackled-up, locked-up, knocked-down, held-down, put-down descendant of a society in Africa, which some archaeologists and other scholars believe was the cradle of civilization. At one time, long before Europe emerged from the dark ages, Africa was the pillar of advanced civilizations.

African civilizations charted the stars, built the pyramids, created written languages, established the calendar as we now know it, and developed networks of world trade as early as 4,000 B.C. With this rich and vibrant African heritage, African-American men have contributed greatly to our community and to the world. It is this innate truth as to who he is and a faith in God that will allow black men to be the pillars of physical and emotional strength that black women and children need.

Many African-American men have played important roles in the training of their children, not only in the past but also today. In the majority of instances, this has been done with very little material wealth with which to be secure, confident, and proud. One conclusion to be drawn from this fact is that, when an African-American man has a secure sense of who he is, he can have a powerful and positive impact on his community and on society in general.

There is a remarkable contrast in these two perspectives. One shows the African-American man disconnected from his heritage with little or no sense of who he is, therefore having no positive contribution to make toward supporting bridging efforts. The other shows the African-American man connected to his rich and vibrant heritage, thereby having a secure sense of who he is. His positive contributions are essential to the African-American community at large.

Look around our community, and you will likely see among black males a significant decrease of self-awareness and an increase in criminal activities (especially violent crimes perpetrated on one another), a high mortality rate (suicide, homicide, and abortion or infant deaths), and the breakdown of the family. Your conclusion based on what you witness may very well be closely aligned with how those negative statistics reflected the status of the black male.

However, in spite of those negative statistics and negative facts, do not believe that African-Americans have survived years of atrocities only to be relegated to a state of derogation and despair. Remember who you are and to Whom you belong! Whenever the African-American man recognizes who he is (a tower of strength) and to Whom he belongs (Almighty God), then his strength can be used as a pillar and his faith in God as mortar for rebuilding his community.

It is critical that black men return to faith in God as their heavenly Father, His Son Jesus as Savior, the Holy Spirit as the teacher and empowerer, and to a belief in family values. The foundation for rebuilding our African-American community lies within the African-American family. To rebuild the family is to rebuild the community.

Rebuilding the Community

Years ago, the black family was the backbone of our community. You did not hear about a high divorce rate or of very many black men fathering children, then abandoning them in the days before World War II. The black family was the black man's support. He depended on it for strength, and the family depended on him for their strength. It was, and should still be, a conjoined unit. In most cases today, however, the black family unit is either falling apart or non-existent in large numbers within the community at large.

In instances where the family has fallen apart, the black man often finds himself confused and lost to at least a certain extent. Many times, there is no sense of "belonging" anywhere. As a result, this sense of not belonging is very evident in the behavior of our children today. *Even when marriages fail despite a good struggle to maintain them, a black man should be an important part of his children's* upbringing, both financially and emotionally. *Men, it is never too late to get involved with your children's lives!*

This is also important in the cases of those men who have fathered children out of wedlock. Children need to know they are loved. If they do not know their parents love them, their lives may be irreversibly damaged. The greatest challenge, if we are to survive, is to teach our children love and good moral values.

The black man needs to realize that his existence and value lies in his ability to love, teach, and pass on his strength to his children. Brothers, we must understand that *to give is to live.* In order to strengthen our community at large and our individual communities specifically, we must bridge some of the gaps. It is critical that we give of ourselves to our children.

Everyone can do something.

Every person has something to contribute toward building up the black community, no matter where he or she lives or works. For example, the very young mother who did not finish high school can share with other young girls her own hardships and experiences. Having a baby at a young age often loses its appeal when a girl realizes how difficult it really will be and how much she will be giving up, both presently and in the future.

The brother recently released from jail also has a powerful testimony to give to young black males headed down the wrong path, the one he just took. Learning what it is like to spend years of your life in prison from someone who has lived through that experience might turn someone else's life around. The entire community should be working to improve its condition.

Particularly, those blacks who have achieved a high level of success should not forget how they got there. The black community is like a pyramid. The affluent/successful African-Americans could not have reached their respective levels of success, if the way had not been paved for them. Many people have the attitude that "I made it on my own!" They need to stop and reflect on *why* they were able to "make it" on their own.

If it had not been for our (collectively *our*) forefathers dying in the streets for their own and subsequent generations' rights to attend school, go to college, obtain jobs in white America, or even to be able to vote, those presently successful individuals more than likely would be unemployed or underemployed, no matter how smart they are Instead of trying to separate themselves from the underprivileged and undereducated blacks, successful blacks should be willing to reach back and help someone else. To be truly successful and have self-gratification, a person must reach out and help someone.

Successful African-Americans should become pioneers in the effort of reaching back in our collective community and helping those who are underprivileged and undereducated. Although some blacks feel uncomfortable talking to those who have achieved a greater level of success in his society, one-on-one relationships can break down those barriers. Regardless of a person's socio-economic status, he or she has something to contribute.

Use your imagination:

• Call a local school and ask how to become involved in tutoring.

• Join a local volunteer organization working in the community.

• Offer to speak to youth in schools or community centers on motivating or informative topics within your experience.

It may be time, it may be financial support, it may be any of a long list of possibilities — but it should be something. If each person were just to adopt one person and take that person on as a prodigy, the results could be astronomical. Children as well as adults, need to have positive role models. Any person can foster a relationship with someone who may benefit from his or her assistance through churches, community organizations, or other creative activities.

The present violence we see increasing in our children has its roots in what they see on television, witness in their schools, hear on the radio, see in the community, and/or are taught in their homes. Those things play a large part in the development of our children.

Recently, I had the opportunity to take part in my church's prison ministry. During a visit to the Memphis Correction Center, I heard a fourteen-year-old African-American youth respond to a question by an adult inmate on why the youth was incarcerated.

The youth answered as proudly as if it were a badge of honor, "I committed murder-one and armed robbery."

This young man has not only thrown his own life away but has taken someone else's life and apparently "wears" his deed as a badge of honor. He is recognized by his peers as having "done something grand." Some juveniles look upon committing a vicious or horrible crime as a "rite of passage" from youth, an initiation into manhood.

Is this type of behavior perpetuated by our adults? We have laws which condemn crimes against society, and the Bible teaches us that we have no right to take the life of another human being. It is wrong both spiritually and legally. However, in American society at large, the negative news and entertainment media have desensitized us to the point where violent behavior is accepted. Such acceptance by adults tells our children that it is okay to commit a crime or take a life.

As adults, we should practice what we preach. If we want our children to live moral lives, then we should lead by example. We should begin to live out morality, responsibility, self-worth, and love in front of them, as well as teach these things to our children.

A storm is coming.

We all see a storm coming. Government is changing. Are we going to be a foolish people or a wise people in preparing for that storm? Government is attempting to abolish affirmative action.

The national budget crisis also will have a major impact on the African-American community. The government is a major employer of African-Americans. Major reforms in welfare and Medicare will have a greater negative impact on blacks because of the disproportionate numbers involved in those programs compared to other races.

We need to begin now to prepare for the tremendous changes that are coming. We cannot simply let this storm occur and "hope for the best." If the government is going to change its operations, then we had better begin to prepare our community to be more self-sufficient. Here are some of the things we need or need to do:

We need more entrepreneurs.

We need more brothers who want to go to college and not to jail.

We need to stop the pattern of "babies having babies."

We need systems in place to ensure the transition for welfare recipients into the private sector to be as smooth as possible — things such as training programs and job-placement assistance.

We need reduced-cost, quality-care centers where children can be safely looked after while parents go to work.

We need assistance in teaching young people how to present themselves and how to find employment.

For many, welfare has been a way of life, something taken for granted. Their mothers and grandmothers were on welfare. Any assistance should not be such that the ones we are trying to help simply become "co-dependent" on something else. Any assistance should be designed to encourage those on welfare to stand on their own feet, not on government or societal programs.

In light of the current climate in government, we *can* do something for ourselves.

[1]*Webster's New World Dictionary of American English*, Third College Edition, (New York: Simon & Schuster, 1988), p. 282.

[2]*Source Book of Criminal Justice Statistics*, Bureau of Justice Statistics, 1994.

[3]"Fact Sheet," (Virginia Beach: Christian Broadcasting Network), November 29, 1995, issue.

Economic Support for
Our Community
by A. Maria Newsome, M.D.

The importance of blacks making a conscious effort to spend more of their money with African-American businesses cannot be overstated.

Economic empowerment in the black community could undo many strongholds that presently prevent us as a whole from enjoying "the American dream." It was not that long ago that blacks suffered tremendous humiliation and, often, even physical abuse during "sit-ins" and other demonstrations aimed at gaining true equality for African-Americans. Many white establishments refused to serve blacks or relegated them to inferior accommodations and service.

Photographs and films testify of blacks and even whites who joined in the civil rights struggle sitting at lunch counters in the 60s while white racists poured ketchup, hot coffee, and other food items over their heads. That history is not ancient; it was not long ago when this happened.

Going even further back in history, there were centuries of time during which blacks could not even dream of owning their own businesses and being their own bosses in America. All they could focus on was staying alive from day to day and enduring the unthinkable hardship of slavery and, later, segregation with the many ills which it caused.

Even today, many African-Americans have difficulty obtaining bank loans to open their own businesses. Numerous reports have shown that many of this nation's lending institutions do not lend money on an equal basis to whites and blacks, although the applicants may have similar backgrounds and similar abilities to repay the loans.

When one considers the tremendous struggle the black race has been through — and continues to go through — in order to establish its own economic stronghold in this country, there is no excuse for blacks refusing to patronize businesses owned by other blacks.

Many contemporary blacks have blocked out the knowledge of this ongoing struggle from their everyday thinking. African-Americans have not yet overcome, although some individual members of the black community believe they have and have no desire to help other blacks attain equality.

Some prefer to patronize a major supermarket five minutes away rather than drive ten minutes to a smaller, black-owned grocery store. Others prefer to drive all the way across town to shop at a large mall or department store rather than to shop at the minority-owned shop on the corner.

Principle Should Outweigh Money

Of course, major chains can purchase goods cheaper than small stores can, whether it is groceries, clothing, or furniture. However, sometimes principle should far outweigh dollars and cents, and this is one of those instances. If a can of beans costs five cents more at the local store, so what?

How many people of other races drive into black neighborhoods to shop at black stores?

How many blacks drive out of the black community to shop at non-minority owned businesses?

If we continue to turn our backs on our own businesses, more and more will have to close, taking with them some of the few existing jobs. We are literally fighting for our economic lives in this area. Because we are not being lynched for standing up for our rights, as was the case with the electoral process, many blacks do not realize this is as serious a struggle.

Today, we are not afraid to voice our opinions for fear a bullet might pierce the living room window. We are not spit upon and humiliated for attempting to be self-respecting citizens. We are not forced to take any dehumanizing, low-paying job just to buy food. And, we are not treating each other with any semblance of respect for the vast sacrifices our ancestors made in order for us to have the rights and privileges we now enjoy.

If black Americans sought out black-owned businesses and made a concerted effort to spend a significant portion of their income with these establishments, we could bring a great deal of healing to our land.

Patronizing the small businessman helps him create jobs for others. Also, the more volume stores do, the more they can lower their prices. The more people who are gainfully employed, the fewer will be committing crimes, suffering from simple medical illness for lack of money to see a doctor, and suffering a lack of self-worth along with countless other negative influences that foster unhappiness and despair.

This is not to say that we should spend all of our income at black businesses. The point is that, as we spend billions of dollars each year as a whole, we must not forget to support our own community. We cannot count on anyone else to do what we refuse to do for ourselves.

Instead of ostracizing African-American establishments, we should be dedicated to discussing problems with management if there is a problem with shopping in a particular store. This is true, no matter whether the store is owned by a black or by a member of another race.

It is not fair to management to withhold our business and talk about the establishment rather than to make a complaint to the proper official and give him or her an opportunity to address whatever problem we have.

There are many avenues one can pursue to find out what businesses are black-owned in a given city or town.

Some cities have a phone directory of black businesses, and some churches have similar directories. Even word of mouth can be a very powerful advertising tool. When we find black businesses, we should tell our friends and family members about them.

If a black-owned store is not able to carry a large inventory, the helpful procedure would be to at least look there first. Then, if the item is not available, go to a larger store or a shopping mall. Although that may mean two trips instead of one, is it not worth a little sacrifice to help accomplish economic empowerment for our race?

Whenever we see newscasts of young black males being arrested for stealing, dealing drugs, or crimes of violence, we ought to remember that, as blacks, we are doing little to provide jobs for those youths. We are *all* responsible for the present state of black America, not just whites.

Instead of crying about what "the white man" has done *to* us and is doing, we need to be busy doing things *for* ourselves. If we spent all that negative energy voting and building up our own communities, racists could no longer have much of an impact upon us.

We would have our own economic stronghold, our own political power, hopefully to work with men and women of all races, but even in those circumstances where this is not possible, we should not have to do without.

How do we get organized in supporting black businesses?

I suggest making a list of how we spend our income, then find out which of these expenses could be handled by a black-owned business in our individual communities. There even are black-owned long distance companies such as *International Telecom* (1-800-787-5200) that offer quality long distance service at competitive prices.

Using this example alone, if 10 percent of blacks signed up with this one company, that would put a tremendous amount of revenue into a black-owned business, thus not only strengthening it but allowing it to grow and create new jobs. This is only one of countless examples of how blacks could use black-owned businesses for things which they purchase every day.

In conclusion, as African-Americans, we must seek out and support black-owned businesses *if we want our communities to flourish*. This issue is not even debatable as to its advisability or importance. Unfortunately, we presently turn our backs on our own for the most part, pouring billions of dollars into companies not committed to uplifting our race.

We need to change, and we need to change now, before the gap between blacks and whites — as well as between black "haves" and "have-nots" — grows beyond repair.

If our African-American community foundation is destroyed, what can we do? We can do a whole lot: *We can rebuild it!*